THE ART OF POSITIVE THINKING

THE 7 MOST POWERFUL BENEFITS OF THINKING POSITIVE EVERYDAY

THE POSITIVE MIND
BOOK 2

BRYANSCOTT PARKER

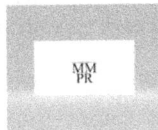

MM
PR

❀ Created with Vellum

CONTENTS

INTRODUCTION

The Art of Positive Thinking

…is rich in its own power source of positive energy. And positive energy is written into our DNA.

I imagine positive thinking as a master dance routine that I choreograph to perfection. Or, positive thinking is the display of a magnificent arrangement of colors, art materials and designs in a masterpiece of artwork; such as the frescos of the Sistine Chapel, designed and painted by the great artist, Michelangelo.

There is something dynamic in the phrase, '*The Art of.*'

This phrase brings out ideas of awe inspiring moments of creativity under the brilliance of the sparkling guiding light of life. And within each one of us this uniqueness exists.

"The essence of 'the art of the positive thinking philosophy' is based in the constructive use of the powers of the mind to create a desired reality." BRYANSCOTT PARKER

But having a positive thinking mindset and being positive everyday does not mean you will be happy and contented in spirit at all times. The philosophy of positive thinking teaches you how to accept every challenge of life. It teaches you to have the confidence of knowing that in your spirit you will overcome all negative outcomes. And you live with continued hope that all your tomorrows can be positive.

Using sincere positive efforts in every situation will create within you, true feelings of joy and satisfaction for all of your life's experiences. And these results are from having the knowledge of a positive thinking mindset.

The Art of Positive Thinking gives you the powers of thinking positive everyday. There is a natural enjoyment in living a positive thinking lifestyle.

Embrace the art of positive thinking with the understanding that everything, every situation, every emotional issue has a beginning, start date and an expiration, end date. And because everything will pass there is never a need or a time to resort to negative thinking or to becoming a negative person. Today, positive thinking philosophies are taught as a necessary mindset for true success in our personal and business lives. Positive thinking should be a course curriculum taught to our children beginning in the grades of elementary school.

The Art of Positive Thinking in 7 chapters shares with you the 7 most powerful benefits of thinking positive everyday.

1. Develop a Genuine *Peace of Mind* with minimal effort.

2. Acquire *Knowledge and Wisdom* everyday.

3. Live with greater *Self-Confidence* making better decisions.

4. Make ***Real Accomplishments*** routinely.

5. Enjoy ***Love & Peace*** with family & friends.

6. Have true ***Love of Self.***

7. Receive ***Personal Happiness*** everyday.

It is pure positive thinking to believe in yourself.

It is positive to believe that you can figure it out no matter what your circumstances may be. Believe, that if you don't have the answers now you will find the answers: They will come. It is better to believe in yourself than not to believe in yourself. Faith begets more faith and faith is inner strength and power.

Positive thinking has its beginnings. Its' roots are from the designer of the human mind: our Creator*.

Follow the information shared in this book. Learn how to gain unlimited access to your thinking mind. Everyday, utilize your naturally positive thinking energies given to all of us at birth.

Create a *'Masterpiece'* for your life and style of living.

Accept the concept...*The Art of Positive Thinking,*...today!

---

* 2Timothy 1:7. For God has not given us a spirit of fear, but of power and of love and of a sound mind.

1

GENUINE PEACE OF MIND

The positivity of the 'Big Bang'

W hen there was nothing…Bang! God created something with His all mighty powers of positive energy.

The "Big Bang Theory" is a widely held belief of the scientific explanation of how our Universe was formed approximately 13.8 billion years ago.

The theory says that at a certain precise moment in time, enormously extreme heat coming from a dense singular object created a cataclysmic explosion that expanded creating an outer space. And as everything cooled from the explosion, the formation of all the heavens and the earth were created.

I accept this theory for lack of any other proof otherwise to explain our existence. But I have a distinct caveat to this idea. The cause of the 'Big Bang' is from the design of our Creator. He designed the massive energy explosion of the Big Bang. The results are the creations of the galaxies, planets, and stars. And the formation for the creation of life as we know it.

The same positive energy coming out of the Big Bang is who and what we are made of today.

Scientific research discoveries of today reveal that we are made of the same elements as the materials of space; the elements that make up the stars in our skies. It has been researched and recorded that there are trace elements of these same materials found in space are in our human DNA. *

All the energies of the universe are from the beginning; the creation of time. And this same positive energy force is replicated over and over again in the intelligent design of each and every one of us as human beings. We are physically endowed from our birth with pure positive energy to overcome every obstacle life may bring. Our principle positive energy forces do not contain one negative energy source for self destruction. When we stay focused on this principle we are continuously reminded that we have the strengths and energies of a positive force to challenge and defeat any negative interference.

When we examine the procreation process of human beings, animals and plants, we see specific instructions of positive energy directives written into the DNA. Positive energy DNA is found in all life forms of every species for survival, self-defense and procreation.

Our bodies perform multiple functions without our mental consciousness or instructions. The heart pumps, the eyes see, the ears hear, the nose smells, the lungs breathe, the feet step, the hands

---

* See Resources: 1. All of the bases in DNA and RNA have now been found in meteorites

2. Thrilling New Evidence Suggests Earth's Life Came from Space.

grab, the legs stand, the arms hold; and the head nods while the brain inside thinks. These are all wired DNA positive functions of the human body. Many of these functions are also found in plant and animal life.

And within the DNA are scripts for the essential regeneration processes of our skin & hair cells and body organs; all with magnificent self healing properties: all functioning without our mental instructions - written into our DNA. We fall down and get skin scrapes, sprains and bruises. Most often if not severe, we self heal, self repair without the need of any medical attention. And when the fall down or skin scrape is severe the body's auto-immune system kicks in to take certain life sustaining measures. For example, without your instruction or intervention an internal adrenaline delivery is given to the body in the event of a bad allergic reaction to a certain food or chemical. The body is positively designed to protect itself with life saving emergency instructions written into our DNA.

The point I am making here is that we are all 'positive wired' for a positive living life from our beginnings. The powers of our human creation are from the same positive energy forces of the Big Bang. And positive energy is naturally in our DNA.

Examine who we are today and measure just how long the World and the creation of the human race has existed and continues to exist. Isn't it our assigned positive initiatives and positive reinforcements contained within our DNA that continues to sustain us? We are designed to be positive thinking human beings without any negative DNA. We have been naturally gifted by our Creator to have the full force of positive thinking energy from birth. *

---

* NKJV 2 Timothy 1:7
   "For God has not given us a spirit of fear, but of power and of love and of a sound mind."

Consider these positive directives. To consummate the birth of a child a single male sperm will aggressively travel on its way to successfully find the female ovum (egg) creating the zygote within the womb of a woman. The positive powers of the male sperm connecting with the female egg inside the womb is the fertilization process needed to bring forth the creation of a child. Only positive energy can create an offspring. Each and every one of us is born from this pure positive energy: And to remain positive energy until the day we die.

It is said that the spirit lives on after the body is gone. Then surely the positive energy we are granted at birth remains in the spirit that lives on…for eternity: So, as it is written.

How the negatives are created and survive

It is our experiences of living life that creates the negative energy in our lives.

Thinking negative thoughts produces our negative behaviors. And our initial negative thoughts are often influenced by our many cognitive distortions.* These distortions enhance and encourage the negative thinking to continue.

But the positive energy forces given to us at birth are still present inside of us. Even though we choose the negative thoughts we think and produce negative behaviors, we can choose not to accept our negative thoughts: We can be redeemed.

We have the power and ability to call on our positive thinking energy whenever we need it. And when we call out to our positive thinking we create the power to remove the negative thinking thoughts.

---

*   See Resources - 15 Cognitive Distortions to Blame for Negative Thinking.

It is because of our positive energy DNA makeup that we are alive and continue to exist is. Each human body is self-contained having a positive energy source (like a battery) that works on auto-pilot.

With the natural functions of the mind to overthink, mixed with our cognitive distortions we create reasons to question our learned positive beliefs. And by questioning the positives we already know, we start to rely on the negatives. Here is where we easily fall into negative thinking behavior patterns. Combine needless overthinking with any one of your cognitive distortions and this all becomes the mental clutter that clogs the minds' positive thinking processes. And these clogging events do the following:

- Generate more overthinking of negative issues creating more negative thought patterns;
- Block the natural response powers of our positive energies to evict our negative thoughts and
- Extend the residential lease on our negative thinking thought patterns so that the negative thoughts remain; blocking the positive thinking thoughts.

These negative thinking behavior patterns become our 'calling cards,' our identities, for life. The consummate liars. The cheaters and the haters who have no respect for themselves and anyone else because they are lost in their beliefs of the powers of their negativity. Our negative thoughts create the negative identities that we follow and admire: Con artists, grifters, liars and cheaters. We openly allow them to dominate our thinking thoughts.

The worst of it all is that this 'circus' of negative thinking is passed on from generation to generation through traditions that allow the negativism to settle in and become part of our culture. Each day is an uphill battle fighting the inherited generational negatives compounded with the daily negatives. And you personally, may not be the one who is creating the negatives. For certain it is the stimulus of our society teaching all of us to accept our negative thoughts as normal. Our cultural societies knowingly or unknowingly use our traditional celebrations as the hidden delivery vehicle for our blind acceptance of our most dangerous negatives:

- jealousy,
- hate and
- deceit.

Without sufficient help and instruction we fall into allowing our negative thinking activity to become part of our daily lifestyle.

In the overthinking of our problems, often due to cognitive distortion behaviors we accept the negative thoughts as the best answers and solutions to our problems. With the acceptance of our cognitive distortions we throw out the truths of the positives we were once taught to believe in. We now mentally entertain and accept our negatives. We embrace and rename our negative behaviors, celebrating them as our newly named positive behavior influencers. To our detriment we openly give strength to negative thoughts and negative persons not realizing we are designing our own self destruction. We applaud the villains, con men and deceivers in our societies as heroes. We, "Follow the yellow brick road," but not to the wisdom of 'OZ' but to the self-destructive desires of lust, greed and deception.

It is time to reorganize our thinking patterns and create a positive thinking mindset that can identify our negative thoughts and prevent our negative behaviors.

The positive thinking mind

Positive thinking is about setting your mind on having an optimistic viewpoint about all things in life. With the knowledge of positive thinking you learn to develop the necessary skills and abilities to be prepared for whatever may happen throughout your lifetime: Good and bad.

We can't see into the future but with a positive thinking mindset we are hopeful to be mentally prepared for the future as it comes. The combined aspects of positive thinking help to form a genuine inner peace. The acceptance of positive thinking acknowledges the following:

- Knowing that you will be resilient in a crisis moment of time.
- Forever ready and available to accept the necessary changes of life.
- Never to lose faith in yourself.

There's an expression that says,"Where there is a will, there is a way." This expression is part of the framework, a cornerstone of the concepts of a positive thinking mindset.

The majority of the negative issues we are challenged with everyday are of our own making. Our thinking of negative thoughts helps to create our poor decision making. And don't forget the influences of self inflicted cognitive distortions.

If we watch our thinking and monitor our thoughts we will find opportunities to design our desired destinies that would include creating a genuine peace of mind.

Becoming more aware of your immediate thought patterns can help you understand the reasons for your emotions and your behaviors.

All reactions in all situations demonstrate certain thought patterns that contribute to overthinking that causes stress, anxiety and needless worry. And more negative thinking follows the overthinking, creating a cycle of more needless worry leading to stress.

Become mindful to pay closer attention to your thinking thoughts. Identify where a thought pattern change is needed. Here is where you can learn to break the cycle of negative thinking and negative behaviors. This is how you reach your inner peace of mind: by breaking the mental cycles of negativity.

As a point of reference to our cycles of negativity, consider taking on the challenge of reducing the amount of annual traditional celebrations you attend. Many of our traditional annual celebrations systemically encourage socially accepted negative thinking behaviors of abusing alcohol and using drugs. This will be a tough challenge for many people because they eagerly look forward to having their traditional celebrations in this manner. But for certain these are the 'entry points' and 'danger zones' that promulgate our historic negative thinking and bad behaviors.

Obtaining a genuine peace of mind for life will remain elusive for the masses of people because of their reasoning and blind acceptance for their annual traditional celebrations.

What is a mindset?

Your mindset is the way you think to come to conclusions and decisions based on your core set of values: The things you have a strong belief in that cause you to react in your own particular way. This is your mindset. It's your unique way of how you think about the things of life.

And by personal desire everyone has a mindset that is either

- fixed and stable in its beliefs with no desire for change, or

- a progressively open mindset willing to change as needed.

" This is how I was born. This is who I am and I can't change it. " Most people are of this mind, set in stone; a stable and fixed mindset. They literally avoid making any changes outside of their personality and they accept their negative attributes with some sort of vague and shadowy pride. They establish a mentally conscious apex to their thinking that says:

"If I don't try it I can't fail at it. So why bother?" This type of mindset creates grand opportunities for negative overthinking.

The other mindset is where a person takes a progressively open thinking position and project an attitude that says;

"There is nothing I can't learn if I truly want to know about it. Each challenge is a new and rewarding experience for me. I will try because I know I will learn something."

This type of mindset accepts positive thinking as a valuable tool to help them make daily and consistent improvements in their lives.

Developing a positive thinking mindset

To have a positive thinking mindset that brings lifelong rewards with a genuine peace of mind you must create and establish parameters for your everyday living.

Your core set of values must include these elements to develop a positive thinking mindset for your life.

1. Think right toward all people. If you sincerely want to live in a positive thinking mindset that gives you happiness everyday, you must think right toward all people. View the public domain of all people as regular, normally nice people who are prone to make mistakes (just like you) because that's how life is.

2. Give a daily hug to your loved ones. Hugging someone is a double treat because both the 'hugger' and the 'huggie' receive the benefits. Hugging allows our oxytocin's to 'percolate.'

3. Find ways to say "I love you," more often than not.

4. Acquire the qualities of a good person. Be honest and sincere with everyone you know and greet.

5. No cheating. No lies. Avoid mischievous and sneaky behaviors.

6. Look for good character traits in other people and reward them by showing some form of appreciation like saying "Thank you for your kindness" or "Thank you for your kind words." Pass it on... Pay it forward.

7. Have no fears. Learn to live without fears of anything. Being fearless actually eliminates many stressful and worrisome situations like job interviews, taking tests, or meeting new people. Be and feel confident that no matter the outcome you will live another day for another chance at the 'good life.'

8. Remain optimistic at all times. When you feel the senses of your positive powers getting low, get recharged! Continue to be positive. Stay aware of your positivity alert indicators. Life can be a drain at times and you must remember to power back up! Get to your personal library of positive thinking self-help materials and read again for reinforcements.

9. Start an exercise routine that can be as simple as taking a brisk walk everyday.

10. Stay in good physical shape by eating only healthy foods. Don't ignore this part of your program because it is one of the most important. Ask yourself, "Where is the benefit in improving my mental thinking if I ignore my physical condition?" You must eat healthy. Make this a solid boundary and your mind will reward

you greatly with a good feeling body and a good looking body too.

11. Get to bed early for a good nights' sleep every night.

12. Be forgiving. Accept the fact that no one is perfect and we all need forgiveness and a second chance. Sometimes a third chance or more.

13. Show genuine gratitude for the blessings you have received by sharing sincere empathy for those who have less than you.

14. Vigorously resist the mental urges of random overthinking. Focus your time wisely to avoid prattle.

> *"Learn to live to get the best out of the most of your life."*
> BRYANSCOTT PARKER

POSITIVE THINKING BREEDS peace of mind

Here are a few principle personality traits to acquire to achieve positive thinking that leads to a genuine peace of mind.

- Empty your mind of all negative thinking thoughts as soon as they appear.
- Be self-aware at all times. Know where you are, know where you are going.
- Maintain focus to stay in control of your emotions and behavior in response to negative thoughts and negative situations.
- Be conscious and respectful of the gifts of nature. Be mindful of your surroundings.
- Accept yourself for who you are. Give value to yourself.

- Reflect gratitude for all the good you are blessed with.
- Live your passion for life. Identify your purpose; something you truly enjoy that motivates you and gives you a positive sense of direction for your life.
- Release all your negatives.

If you are feeling completely out of sorts and you are having a hard time finding any inner peace, please reach out for professional support counseling. They have the talent to help you manage your way through the challenges to finding peace.

FIND a quiet place for your peace

Everyday go to your quiet place to simply sit, using the time to think and become aware of your thinking thoughts. Literally, within your mind identify when you are thinking negatively or and positively. Make a list of what causes the negative thinking and what causes the positive thinking to occur. With this information you can see what activity is bringing on the negative thoughts that need to be eliminated. Watch for distortions in your thinking such as:

- blaming others for your faults;
- always thinking you are right and
- making useless unverifiable excuses

These are just a few of the cognitive distortions our mind creates to avoid positive thinking.

Begin a system of actually choosing the positive thoughts you need to achieve your goals. Use affirmations and prayer to help build a mental platform that will help you to create more positive thinking thoughts. (Using affirmations and prayer is further discussed in Chapter 3.)

The process of choosing your thoughts is the first step to helping develop and create a positive thinking platform for a positive thinking mindset. In every thinking situation identify the words and actions you associate with the positive thinking thoughts and the negative thinking thoughts. Validate each negative thought as fact or fiction. Retain the positive ideas that can be applied and used later. Throw out the negatives.

Get vigilant and completely aware of what it is you are actually thinking. This activity will feel strange at first but in time you will automatically become more aware of identifying your thinking thoughts.

Find your quiet place. Go there just to think about your thoughts.

Move forward toward your goal: To have a positive thinking mindset for your life.

MAKE the positive change

Throughout history it has been the people with positive attitudes and the positive thinking mindsets that have ruled the World. And it is positive minded people who are ruling the World today. Whether or not they have the right doctrine may be at question but nonetheless it is the positive thinking people who are in charge.

You want to be positive because positive energy is what gets life going and keeps it going. It is said that salespeople make the world go around because of their abilities to sell products. The manufacturer makes the product. But it does take a salesperson to sell the product. There's the positive movement. This is the positive energy that makes life evolve in the business world.

The mind is vast in its purposes. While it controls and maintains all of our necessary body functions it keeps us connected to all of nature and with each other as one people.

The thinking of thoughts, positive and negative are generated in the mind. If negative thinking thoughts can produce negative activity then let's all learn the art of positive thinking for good. Let's eliminate negative thinking all together.

People with a positive thinking mindset develop coping skills to do the following:

- Avoid and reduce overthinking
- Stop needless worrying; eliminating stress
- Experience less depression; no anxiety
- Improve psychological analytical skills
- Develop stronger resistance to the common cold and flu symptoms
- Live more productive lives due to better physical well-being
- Live longer lives
- Learn to experience life one day at a time
- Share valuable time with their loved ones

A Positive thinking mindset tells us:

- There is nothing wrong that can't be fixed. And if it can't be fixed we will find another way to work things out.
- There is no failure. Whatever the outcome of the situation, it can and will be accepted as it is to learn from the experience.
- Everything happens in life for its own reasons and purposes.
- Accept the facts that life offers no guarantees of success. None. No guarantees!

So what are you waiting for?

Those of us who are proclaimed positive thinkers have faith and belief in ourselves. And we generally make good decisions. We don't succeed at every moment or at every outing. But we consistently succeed most of the time by simply living each day to the best of our positive abilities; one day at a time. We can't control all the negative events that will happen in life. But we can control our responses to all events to create a better outcome.

Think positive first. Use your natural abilities of positive thinking. It's in your DNA.

Be honest with the truth

The root word of truth is 'true.' The Merriam-Webster dictionary says that if something is true it is;

- 1. in accordance with fact or reality;
- 2. accurate or exact;
- 3. loyal or faithful;
- 4. honest.

Truth, as defined is;

- 1. the quality or state of being true;
- 2. that which is true in accordance with fact or reality;
- 3. a fact or belief that is accepted as true.

My interpretation; the most logical conclusion of a thought is the truth.

One of the basic foundations needed for achieving a positive thinking mindset is a dedication and commitment to knowing and respecting the truths contained in all the areas of life. It is important to be receptive and honest with the truth as it is written. If you keep an honest and positive outlook on your life you will create a healthy mental attitude. A healthy mental attitude generates more positive energy.

Life is the experiences of the actual moments in time as they happen: This is life. Yesterday has gone. Tomorrow is a projection. Actual life and living is only in the moments of our here and now: today.

The truth is so vitally important to know and understand at all times because time itself, is fleeting. And all life is made of time. Don't waste your time hesitating to accept the truths of life. Don't waste your precious time with untruths and lies. There will be no genuine peace of mind in your life if you entertain lies and untruths.

As life exists purely one day at a time, practice filling each day with positive thinking thoughts and positive actions. Be honest with yourself. In time you will have a more durable positive thinking mindset that works for you all the time.

Thinking positively everyday, you can live your life to the highest point of your living with joy and happiness one day at a time. This is the apex of life.

A benefit of having peace of mind

Here is a real life event that most likely happens all the time, somewhere.

You are fired or terminated from your job unexpectedly. Because you know your job skills, abilities and your self worth, you immediately tell yourself that you will be ok.

After the initial shock of the job loss wears off, energy from your positive thinking mindset kicks in. Immediately, the positive thinking processes of your self confidence and self esteem prevent any needless overthinking, worry, stress and anxiety about your sudden job loss. Knowing that you have full confidence is your abilities to find another job you now contemplate if you should stay in the same line of work. Wisely you consider this sudden job loss as a sign. Maybe it's time to make a change; a move forward to advance your career.

Sometimes the unexpected displeasures of life can be a sign of the time to make a life change. And now, you have choices. One of the greatest spices of life is to have options; having choices.

When we remain consistently aware of our true self-worth we can always be flexible and adaptable to nearly every situation as it happens to us. This is having a genuine peace of mind.

MAINTAIN your peace of mind

Bring more definition to your life by determining where you want to be in life.

- What kind of person are you?
- What kind of person do you want to be?
- Where do you fit in?

Literally and physically observe and participate in the things of nature. Visit the 'outdoors' more often. Engage with nature. Gods' gifts to mankind are the animals of the forests and beasts of the seas. Take the time to look in awe of His creations. He has also made for our personal self-enjoyment the love of diamonds, pearls rubies, gold and silver. The pleasures of furs and minks. The fragrances of sweet perfumes and aphrodisiacs, the flavors of wines and nectars of honey and fruits, all for our pleasures. What an awesome God! He loves all of us. The good people and the bad people are His creations.

But acknowledge that your happiness in life is your responsibility. And if you base your happiness on a loving Creator you will be happy most of the time with peace of mind even in days of distress.

Having a genuine peace of mind does not mean you will be happy and content at all times. The process is to create a place in your mind where you can always go to relax from the pressures of life.

Acquiring a genuine peace of mind will come from having a true understanding of the goals you are working to achieve relevant to your life's desires. Whatever your true desires are they must be attainable at a level that you can achieve them. Set goals for yourself that are reachable. Set goals that you can maintain. And then you can enjoy a genuine peace of mind to last your lifetime.

Having a genuine peace of mind is not a pipe dream. Having peace of mind everyday is a life journey.

Plan your thinking wisely. Practice each day to learn to live with a genuine peace of mind, everyday.

CHAPTER 1 RECAP

Genuine Peace of Mind

- The Positivity of the Big Bang
- How the negatives are created and survive
- The positive thinking mind
- What is a mindset?
- Developing a positive thinking mindset

- Positive Thinking breeds peace of mind
- Find a quiet place for your peace
- Make the positive change
- Be honest with the truth
- A benefit of having peace of mind
- Maintain your peace of mind

ACQUIRE KNOWLEDGE AND WISDOM

Knowledge creates wisdom power

The Merriam-Webster Dictionary defines *knowledge* as:

- a(1) : the fact or condition of knowing something with familiarity gained through experience or association.
- (2) : acquaintance with or understanding of a science, art, or technique.
- b(1) : the fact or condition of being aware of something.
- (2) : the range of one's information or understanding.

As we live we learn and acquire knowledge from our living experiences. Knowledge is everything and knowledge is in everything. And just like time, knowledge is fleeting. If you don't use it you can lose it. Every situation creates an opportunity to learn and acquire knowledge.

I share with you a true story of a time in my young life.

Actual knowledge can be learned from something as simple as knowing when and how to cross a heavily traveled city street.

I will always visually remember the day my oldest sister took me by the hand to teach me how to cross a busy street for my first time. It all happened in a small urban city in Connecticut. Our family at that time was my Mom, me and my three brothers and one sister; Angel Rose. I was a middle child on the young end of 4 boys.

We lived on Main Street, one of the busiest main streets in this inner city. The building we lived in was a 3 story, 6 unit brick building with each floor having 2 huge apartments consisting of 4 bedrooms each. Our apartment was on the top floor, front side of the building facing Main Street. At anytime of the day or night you could look out of the window and see the fast moving traffic in both directions down on Main Street. What a scary scene that was for me, an 8 year old. The name of the street itself loomed large in my imagination as a place of commotion and noise. There were sounds of police cars and ambulance sirens screaming and racing up and down the road all day and through the night. At times it seemed to me that Main Street was the only place in the entire world and everything was happening all at once; here on Main Street.

For all the time we had lived on Main Street, for about 2 years up until then, I had no reason or desire to cross over to the other side of Main Street. On the other side was a just a large cemetery that stretched out for at least three city blocks. Fortunately for me the schools we attended were on the same side of the street as our apartment building. I felt very comfortable knowing that I would never have to cross Main Street. Angel Rose, my big sister was three years older than I and she insisted that it was time for me to learn how to cross Main street.

"Give me your hand and just keep walking straight ahead," were her instructions as she grabbed hold of my arm. Full of fear of being

hit by a car as the traffic was so busy I cringed all the way to the other side hearing the screeching tires coming and going on both sides of the four lane road. Angel Rose holding tightly onto my arm had brazenly walked us directly out into the oncoming traffic!

Once we reached the other side she said to me, *"See. They know they better not hit us and they better slow down and stop when they see people crossing the street."*

Yikes! My heart was doing flips all the way to the other side of the road and this was her reasoning for crossing a busy street?I was as scared as petrified fear could ever be. The cars were coming right at us honking their horns while pumping their brakes attempting to slow down to avoid hitting and running us over.

Once we did reach the other side of the street I began to calm down. And then I visualized what could have happened if one of the drivers was not paying attention to the road, smoking a cigarette or just looking in another direction. I asked Angel Rose this question and her response was *"If they hit us they will go to jail."* And I immediately said, *"Yes. And we will be dead!"*

What I learned from this incident, at being just 8 years old was that you don't blindly follow anyone into a dangerous life threatening situation. Even if it is your big sister, Angel Rose. This was an experience for me where I gained two huge pieces of knowledge that day:

- 1. How *not* to cross a busy street and;
- 2. How some people can be totally wrong and possibly dead wrong because of their ways of thinking.

I never crossed another street with my sister. Using this experience I found the best way to cross any street was to simply go to the desig-nated crosswalks, as was taught in school. And if there are no crosswalks and you are caught in the middle of the walkway just patiently wait until there would be no cars coming at all from either direction. The traffic on Main Street did slowdown periodically but you could never anticipate when the slowdown would occur or how long it would last. What a busy street.

In my thinking, I came to the conclusion that whenever crossing any street there exists no need to rush to get to the other side. And that simply crossing a street is never worth the risk of life or loss of limb.

Reflecting back to those times I remember there was an auto insurance commercial that used the theme, *"Always watch out for the other guy."* The commercial was referring to the facts that while you may be driving correctly and safely the 'other guy' (driver) may be intoxicated, smoking a cigarette, looking the other way or just being distracted and not paying attention to the road. Subsequently you could be involved in an accident not of your fault.

Throughout my growing years I thoughtfully applied this theme to other areas of my life because it makes pure positive sense: be aware, stay alert and always consider the other person. Watch out for the other guy in all of life's situations. Stay focused and mindful of what you are doing and where you are going at all times. This was real positive knowledge that I learned from the event of crossing the street with my big sister.

In my later years as a teenager I came to an understanding of my sister's idea of crossing the street was comparable to playing 'Russian Roulette'. Angel Rose was willing to gamble and take poor risks with her life by not considering the possible consequences of her decisions. Reflecting upon this single experience from my childhood, it became a root cause of my acceptance of positive thinking today. I learned to not blindly accept another persons' way of thinking. Study, analyze and verify their actions for reasonableness before making the decision to accept their advice or instructions.

Wisdom

Merriam-Webster Dictionary defines wisdom as;

- a. Ability to discern inner qualities and relationships: INSIGHT;
- b. Good sense: JUDGEMENT;
- c. Generally accepted belief;
- d. Accumulated philosophy or scientific learning: KNOWLEDGE

Wisdom is developed in the mind from years of acquiring positive intelligent knowledge. Wisdom is the actual use of the knowledge you have acquired over time. When we can mentally call upon and receive the solution or remedy to apply to a situation, we have demonstrated acquired wisdom coming from the base of the knowledge we have learned.

Wisdom embodies insight, judgement and knowledge.

THE POWER of words

Here are three poignant quotes taken from a Barnes & Noble email advertising article March 8, 2024 titled, 'The Era of Woman.' The article hi-lights women authors and their views on writing and reading in todays' world.

*"The act of reading outside of your experience increases empathy. It broadens our understanding of humanity and our ideas about who we are and about what we can be."*Jesmyn Ward

"Writing is an extreme privilege but it's also a gift. It's a gift to yourself and it's a gift of giving a story to someone." Amy Tan

"We live in a moment and a culture when reading is really endangered. There's simply no way to write well, though, if you're not reading well." Jennifer Egan

The power of the printed word is immense. Words are our communication vehicles that stimulates our thinking and delivers our thoughts to cause movement in our lives.

When speaking and writing use a more specific word type that can give more depth of meaning to your message. There are certain words that have the power to convey more depth of spirit and feeling than other words. Allow your words to compete for your attention and delivery in your personal conversations and professional discussions. Here's an example.

Compare these two phrases. "time is fleeting" and "time is passing."

Time is passing is conveying that time is moving forward never to return. So the emphasis here is on the forward movement of time. Using the word "fleeting," conveys that time is moving fast and more vividly expresses the need to understand that time is waiting for no one, gone in an instant never to return. The phrase "time is fleeting," conveys more of the actual reality of time moving fast and not just passing.

This word example may be somewhat exaggerated but the point should be clear. Certain words are more expressive than others. Choose your words wisely for better understanding in communicating. By using words that have the power and ability to display your thoughts in a more expressive and definitive way you create within your mind a more rhythmic pattern of talking that will generate a more enhanced and attentive sound to your listening audience.

An increased vocabulary (word count) stimulates the imagination and adds to your intellect that increases your intelligence. With more word ammunitions at your disposal the more creative your positive powers to communicate will be. And the more confident you will be in your speaking.

In your everyday communications and conversations be mindfully aware of the people who use a limited vocabulary to express themselves. Understand this: No one can imagine something if they don't think of it. You don't think about something you can't imagine.

People who use the same general words in verbal and written communications display a limited intellect. There will be no visible growth in their personality or their lifestyle. Those of a limited vocabulary generally have little to offer in conversation and substance.

A strong vocabulary is capable of a healthy and beneficial imagination with huge personal growth potential. The knowledge and use of a multiple word vocabulary easily expands the imagination of possibilities and choices. Having choices is one of the spices of living a good life more abundantly. Add more words to your vocabulary. Your messages delivered through your improved vocabulary become more easily acceptable and even more trustworthy whenever you speak.

It is accepted in many social circles that,

"What you don't know can't hurt you."

But in the true reality of life what you don't know is hurting you if the knowledge you don't know is important to your personal development and an integral part of your career growth. The other side to this statement in response is,

"You would have been or could have been if you had only known."

The more you learn about what you don't know the better you will be equipped to know how to live life more abundantly.

For your benefit make the time to learn what you should and need to know. Read. Study. Grow. Follow the printed word. Words are important and all words matter. The more words in your vocabulary the better communicator you will be to a larger audience of people.

All of us are captivated by certain words, certain phrases and how they are used. Consider the words used to sell products in advertising. The right words mean everything to making a sale.

INCREASE your vocabulary

Share this exercise with family and friends to increase your vocabulary.

One day while having a casual discussion with a few friends inject a new word or two into the conversation. Look for who shows an alertness to the new word and who continues on without any mention of the new word. The friend who asks "What does that mean?" has an awareness principle in their personality. This person has ears to hear and eyes to see. Most likely this person can be taught to learn new things very easily. But if no one in the group asks for the meaning of the new word repeat the word again and ask everyone if they understood the word. This would be a perfect time to share with them the fun and educational benefits of increasing their vocabulary.

Consistently adding new words to your vocabulary is a part of creating and maintaining a positive thinking mindset. I have placed at the end of this book, a Glossary of the more descriptive words I used in writing this book. During Bible study lessons I was advised to have a dictionary at my side while reading. This proved to be an invaluable technique in the process of learning and understanding the material. So I have incorporated the glossary concept into all of my self-help book.

Every word we use identifies and defines our thoughts. The more words you know the more variety of thoughts you will have. The quality of your life can be limited by the imagination of your thoughts. When we can increase our imagination we have the chance to grow further in our thinking giving us the potential ability to improve our living. Adding new words to your vocabulary will magically increase your thinking thoughts which increases your world of imagination. You gain the ability to grow in many new directions when you make it part of your life plan to learn new words everyday. Add to your vocabulary to increase your knowledge that will increase your positive thinking thoughts.

In the Bible, Jesus, speaking to His disciples in explaining the meaning of parables says to them, "He who has eyes, see. He who has ears, hear." When I read these words of instruction my eyes get focused, my ears perk up and I listen more intently. It is a reminder to me to pay attention and to listen more closely for the true meaning of my thoughts and my spoken words.

Everyday make it a priority to become more familiar with new words and terms that help to remind you of your positive thinking. Add power to your day. Add new words to your vocabulary.

Make the positive change

You must be persistent, determined and available for change to achieve your positive goals. A strong and positive thinking mind is forever open to the ideas of change. Accept a personality change as an opportunity for positive mental growth and development.

To achieve lifelong beneficial results, design your daily routines for positive thinking and physical conditioning.

- Set adequate sleep times.
- Exercise your body and
- Maintain a healthy foods diet.

For mental well being…

- Read more!
- Include prayer and meditation with positive affirmations.

Become more self-aware of your strengths and weaknesses. Whatever negative setbacks you may have experienced, research them and reclassify each one as an opportunity to learn something positive about yourself.

Read to learn and grow. Develop your personal cache of self-help materials and books based in the concepts listed here. Acquire the necessary elements of creating a positive thinking mindset library that will be with you for your life's journey. Incorporate these concepts into your daily planning.

- self-mastery
- self-motivation
- self knowledge
- self-correction
- self-development
- self-achievement
- self-gratification
- self-appreciation

Notice the daily planning is focused on 'self.' It is, 'all about you.' You are reading these materials to create a better you.

The printed word is the path to the real truths of the world. And it is foolish to believe that it will be ok to put your faith in someone else's hands to tell you the truths you need to know about living your life. If you don't read for yourself you must wait for someone to tell you what you need to know for your life. Although there are many people who have learned certain things in life without read-ing, it is a poor attitude to refuse or ignore the importance of reading for self-help, self-teaching and personal growth.

Positive self-teaching does require some form of a dedication to reading regularly. Get over the 'hump' if you are 'stuck on a stump' avoiding the benefits of reading.

Reading is fundamental to learning how to live a better life. Your reading must be included in some kind of routine schedule if you intend to succeed at achieving your goals of a positive thinking mindset.

Read with the intent to build a resource library of self-help, self-improvement materials. Having your own library will keep you up to date with easy access to the latest information. It also allows you the pleasures of reading at your leisure.

VISUALIZE your positive change

It is better, much better to believe in yourself than not to believe. Believe that you CAN figure it out. Believe that it is your turn for real happiness and success using your positive thinking energies. Here are a few helpful facts to know about your mind.

- Know that your mind listens to you when you talk.

- Know that your mind works for you.
- Tell your mind what you want it to do.
- RE-MIND yourself regularly that the energy of positive thinking is in your DNA.

Positive thinking is power and there is power in simply thinking positive thoughts. If we dedicate ourselves to our desires to be positive, everything we think and do will reflect that dedication to creating a positive thinking mindset.

Plan your future

In your planning acquire the skill to predict your options and see the end results before you execute your plan.

Whatever your scheduled actions are within your planning, try to predict the ending results before you activate the plan. And be determined to making positive ending results from your planning.

Planning to have a truly positive thinking mindset is more than just thinking positive and reciting positive affirmations daily. As these two functions are very important and necessary, the main events that will cause the positive development of your new positive thinking lifestyle is found in your positive actions based in your actual activities.

- Find positive ways to actually help other people. Especially those who are less fortunate than you. The needy, the homeless, the in-firmed.
- Share some of your quality time with positive thinking people.
- Stay in good physical health by eating healthy foods and exercising.

- Avoid negative thinking thoughts immediately. Replace them with positive thoughts.
- Avoid negative thinking people and negative situations.
- Accept the fact that life happens one day at a time.
- Be self-forgiving and show appreciation for yourself. It is very important to have self love.
- Be kind to yourself every single day!
- Show gratitude and thankfulness to your Creator, in prayer each day.

I have intentionally repeated the following thought for greater emphasis because it is vitally important; but also very easy to implement.

1. Know that it is easier to change your mindset to think positive thoughts than to continue to accept your current negative thinking thoughts. Because the power of positive energy to think positive is in your DNA.

2. It is easier to change to a positive thinking person than to continue to accept the negative thinking encounters you have become so accustomed to accepting. Because the power of positive energy to think positive is already in your DNA.

3. It is easier to change the way you think by changing your thought patterns than to continue to allow negative, stressful, worrisome and anxious thought patterns to continue. Because the power of positive energy to think positive is already in your DNA.

Empty your mind of all negative thoughts immediately. Fill your mind quickly with healthy positive thinking thoughts.

FAITH AND BELIEF

Have faith without seeing.*

Can you prove that the Earth is round? When we look out onto the horizon the Earth appears flat. If you walk the Earth to find an ending we will walk in a circle never finding the ending because the Earth is round. But can you see the earth as round while being on Earth? No. The only way we can physically see the Earth as round would be to fly out into space and physically view the earth from a spaceship. The Earth will alway appear flat to us while here on Earth.

When we look to the horizons we see a straight line. This is an optical illusion that we see everyday. Because the earth is round as a sphere, there is no actual delineation line to find. The horizon that we see is created by the Sun's reflection off the Earth. Because we cannot physically see the entire Earth, it is by faith we live and believe the Earth is round. Although the visual we see is flat, we know from scientific research and historical data that the Earth is round. And the optical illusions of the horizons we see are accepted as delineations.

The Moon and the stars are visible but only scientifically explained. And we believe all that science says about them because we can't go up into space to see them for our own inspection. But they are there and we accept them as such. This is our faith again. Technology has taken us to the moon and outer space where these celestial bodies were identified and verified at a closer range. But it is still our trust in the word of others that we accept and believe these concepts as real.

Obtaining knowledge that creates wisdom is an ongoing task for

---

*   NKJV JOHN 20:29
    Jesus said to him, "Thomas because you have seen Me, you have believed. Blessed are those who have not seen and yet have believed."

life. As we live each day the opportunity to learn something we didn't know yesterday will always exist. And no one person or group of people can know everything there is to know about life.

Also, knowledge is fleeting. What you will learn this year you will forget before next year if you are not using the information.

Accept your life as a journey through time. On this journey you acquire the knowledge you need to continue to exist; one day at a time. Applying the wisdom of knowledge in your daily life increases your enjoyment of the pleasures found in all of life. Using a positive thinking mindset you can rejoice in your abilities to solve your problems as they happen. This is how you avoid overthinking and needless worry using your acquired wisdom of positive thinking.

A very dear friend I had the privilege of knowing, a decorated World War II Veteran said to me, *"Bryanscott, we are just a blip on the spectrum of time. In short order, we are here and then we are gone: Just a blip in time."* In loving memory of my friend, Mr. Buddy Pease.

Everyday be mindful to pay attention to what is happening in your presence. Stay aware of all things within your surroundings. This means the birds, the bees and the trees: God's gifts of nature. Make time to have meaningful conversations with family and friends for intellectually stimulating discussions. Avoid prattle and idle gossip as topics of your conversations. Have talks about many different things that you may have an interest in that express positive values for living life.

As you make mistakes and errors in judgement, accept these errors as lessons learned. Let all your missteps be areas where you can make positive changes that will improve your future growth.

Make real plans for a real future having faith and belief in a positive thinking mindset.

A wisdom moment

Recalling a time from my property management real estate years...

One afternoon while relaxing at home after working the day at one of my two family rental houses, one of my tenants called me to say that her electricity wasn't working and she had no lights. Nonny, a single mom with her 9 year old daughter, Payton was renting the second floor, two bedroom apartment. They had been tenants of mine for two years now. I was at the house earlier that day installing two small basement storm windows.

This two family house, built during the late 1800's was quite stout and sturdy. Built on a solid natural stone rock foundation, it was one of my favorite two family houses I owned at the time. I purchased the property partly for the reason of the stone foundation; even though it showed a slightly wet basement. In doing my due diligence to purchase the property I identified what I needed to do to solve the wet basement issue. When I made my offer to purchase, I requested a reduction to the asking price because of the wet basement. My lower price offer was accepted.

The caveat to the purchase of this two family was that it had a legal third floor one bedroom, kitchen and bath apartment. But there was only one entry/exit and this caused the unit to be illegal to rent out as a separate one bed room unit. But I saw the way to resolve this issue. I would rent the second floor two bedroom unit with the third floor one bedroom apartment as a total package of three bedrooms with additional kitchen and bath. Throughout my time of ownership of the property I did rent the two units together just as I had envisioned when I purchased the property. But at this time, Nonny my second floor tenant did not need three bedrooms. So the third floor apartment was vacant at this time.

It was late in the afternoon and darkness had come to the end of the day. I asked Nonny if she knew where the circuit breakers in the basement was and she replied *"No."* I told her that I could be there in about 30 minutes to restore the lights.

On the way driving to the house I gave myself mental instructions as to what I would need to do to fix whatever the electrical problem was. In my thinking I remembered that I had a conversation with Nonny earlier in the day. She had a male visitor in the apartment at the time and I now remembered that the two of them appeared to be somewhat inebriated. Thinking about that conversation now, I thought it was odd that she made no attempt to introduce her male friend to me. And he seemed to avoid making eye contact with me when I was talking with her. Another observation I made was that Nonny did not own a car and there wasn't a car in the parking lot at that time of her friend's visit other than my truck. This told me that her visitor, simply judging from his appearance and with no other car in the parked in the driveway, that most likely he did not own a car. Nothing major to that thought; just an observation.

I called upon my memory of past tenant actions and responses in certain situations. Quickly I adjusted my thinking and determined that I should be cautious and swift to fix the electrical problem as fast as possible to avoid any personal interactions or possible alter-cations. It was likely Nonny and her friend were still drinking.

The two-family house had two separate entrances to get to the second floor apartment where Nonny lived; The parking lot entrance and a side of the building entrance. The parking lot entrance was a slightly steep and narrow stairwell leading to the apartment entry door. There was one small ceiling light fixture at the top of the stairs to light the stairway. This is the entrance I regularly used when coming from the parking lot or when coming up from the basement to get to the second floor apartment.

Once I had arrived, after going to the basement and resetting the electrical breaker I headed for Nonny's apartment. At that precise moment a loud voice echoed a mental command in my head saying, *"Do not use the parking lot entrance to the second floor; use the side entrance."* In a flash, I become mentally vigilant and alert. I listened to my mind and did exactly as I was instructed: I used the side entrance to the apartment. I opened my eyes wide, perked up my ears to listen intently and proceeded with caution.

Using the side entrance, I went up to the second floor apartment and knocked on the door. When Nonny opened the door I immediately said to her *"It should be ok to turn on the lights."* While I waited in the threshold of the doorway I watched her flick the light switch on the wall. At that moment I could hear her male friend coming into the apartment from the parking lot/stairwell entrance. Once he had entered the apartment and came into the room I noticed he was holding in his right hand a short round stick along side his leg: I considered this just another observation.

The lights to the apartment were now working. Still standing in threshold of the doorway I quickly said goodnight to Nonny and she politely said thank you and I left.

As I was driving home I began recalling the memory of this evenings' event. I thought of Nonny's friend wielding the short stick. Could he have been lying in wait for me on the stairwell at the parking lot entry door anticipating my entry there? For a possible attempt to rob me? The parking lot entry stairwell provides a small enough space where you could trap someone.

I now believe, to this day that the electrical problem Nonny called me for may have been a rouse to lure me to the house for that purpose. My training of mental awareness to stay focused at all times caused my mind to speak to me at the precise moment. And I obeyed immediately.

When we pay attention and consciously observe our surroundings, we get to use acquired knowledge that creates the wisdom to help us improve our everyday living, long into our future.

HAVING trust in others

It is better to have trust in what you read for yourself rather than to have blind trust in what people are telling you.

Before giving your trust to someone consider using the policy advice given by our former President of the United States, Mr. Ronald Reagan; Trust. Then verify. Are the facts valid? Verify the truth in the facts that are given to you.

It is hugely beneficial for every one of us, individually and collectively to embrace goodness, the truth and the law. Allow your acquired knowledge to become your proven wisdom for the benefits of having a better life.

CHAPTER 2 RECAP

Acquire Knowledge and Wisdom

- Knowledge creates wisdom power (ACTUAL EVENT)
- Wisdom
- The power of words
- Increase your vocabulary

- Make the positive change
- Visualize your positive change
- Plan your future
- Faith and belief
- A wisdom moment (ACTUAL EVENT)
- Having trust in others

3

GOOD DECISIONS BUILD CONFIDENCE

It's all in your mind...

This is the paradox we all live with.

"Although the mind creates all of your problems, it is your mind that is also the only thing in charge of solving them." Excerpt from the book, OVERTHINKING? 7 Steps to Finding Peace from Overthinking Stress, Anxiety and Worry; author Bryanscott Parker.

It is our mind that visualizes and makes all choices and decisions in all situations; it is our mind that will bring us through all situations to their end. And if you allow or encourage negative thoughts and negative ideas into your thinking process, for certain your actions will result in negative behaviors.

Strong negative thoughts are a demon force that eliminates the positive thinking choices of our decisions. In our mind the negative thoughts are taking up residency. And over time you eventually start to believe the negatives as your truths - because that's all you have for choices to draw on in making decisions.

Your negative thinking thoughts are reinforced with the help of your cognitive distortions such as:

- You always wanting to be right in a conversation or group discussion;
- You are always jumping to conclusions without the facts or valid reasoning;
- You ignore the positive alternatives in all situations;
- You have a "it's me, me, me" attitude.

These negative mental distortions and others like them create thinking patterns that distract or eliminate our naturally positive thinking patterns.

And on the other side, when we intentionally fill our mind with positive thinking thoughts the mind will produce positive thinking patterns that create positive behavior actions.

When we can identify our cognitive distortions, such as the ones mentioned above, we can learn to override most or all of them simply by using positive thinking affirmations. It really is that simply: And easy. Create the habit of using positive affirmations consistently each time you perceive a negative thought coming. Example:

- I don't have to be right all the time.
- I don't know all the facts - I won't make a decision until I can get more answers to my questions.
- Wait…there could be another way to solve this issue.
- I must accept the facts that other people are important too. It's not always about me.

Remember…Your mind does listen to you when you tell it what to do. Notice how easily it works when you want the 'bad' stuff; the negatives? Well, it works just as easy for the 'good' stuff; the positives. But, because you have accepted the bad for so long it will require more effort to make the change from the bad negatives to the good positives.

We were created with and born of positive energy. And we can call upon our positive thinking energy whenever we choose because it is in our DNA. It is in the mind where we make our decisions based on the choices we have before us. And our choices are stored within our intellect. Here is where all that we know from what we have learned is stored and classified as our facts.

NEGATIVE THOUGHTS ARE LIKE BULLIES.

Have you noticed that once you entertain a negative idea the negative thoughts surrounding that negative idea start to multiply and become negative thinking? And if you don't literally say to yourself *"Stop! That's enough already,"* the negative idea will find a place to hibernate in your mind. There, it waits until you summon it to reoccur for some more negative thinking. Once negative thoughts take up residency in your mind they stay there sucking up all the oxygen in the room leaving very little space for any positive thinking to occur.

Your negative thoughts help to create overthinking issues. They take up the dominant positions in your mind to pop up as the answers and solutions to all of your problems. Confusion, indecision and worry become the daily 'Bill of Fare' for your mind. Until you mentally remove your negative thoughts and replace them with positive thinking thoughts the negatives will not leave you.

But when you fill your mind with positive thoughts that produce positive thinking the negative thoughts will be removed permanently.

FIND confidence in your decision making

The best decisions come from having great choices. Our choices are maintained in our intellect. The intellect is made stronger by adding more knowledge to it. Knowledge is increased from more reading and reading is fundamental to learning.

Making good decisions builds your confidence. It is wise and beneficial to establish a routine of reading positive self-help materials. Positive thinking thoughts build a positive intellect. Having a positive intellect allows you to draw from a better selection of choices in making decisions.

Decision making is a thought driven process.

If our initial thoughts identify the decision to be made is a difficult decision to make, we will generally make a poor decision. Conversely, if we think the decision to be made is easy to decide, we will make a good decision.

The two main influencers to our decision making process are:

- 1. Thinking too fast. Thinking too fast in making a decision can lead to a bad decision. Instinctively we make fast decisions based in our own particular biases that require very little thinking.
- 2. Thinking too slow. Our slow thinking may be intentional where we take the time to make careful considerations of certain factors to help us make the best decision. Slow

thinking requires lots of time and still offers no guarantees of a best decision.

Using a combination of both thinking methods is the wisest choice.

If our thoughts are negative most of the time then we will produce negative decisions most of the time. Consistently making bad decisions indicates low to no self-confidence. Conversely, if our thoughts are positive most of the time then we can expect to make positive decisions most of the time, creating a stronger confidence base.

The 2 most common negative thinking decision making platforms comes from the cognitive distortion behaviors of catastrophizing and all-or-nothing thinking.

When we catastrophize in our thinking we are imagining the worst possible outcome of the situation: "It's gonna be a catastrophe!" Going to this extreme in our thinking can cause the avoidance to make any decision at all. Or make a decision that may not be in our best interest.

All-or-nothing thinking is to view everything with a black or white mentality with no middle ground for further discussion of the situation. This decision making platform doesn't allow for comparisons of the many possible options available to make a more informed decision.

To make better decisions always consider the outcome of all the options that are available. Think of as many possible solutions and answers there may be to help you choose the best decisions. And once you make the decision, follow through and take action. *"Do I go right or left? Is the answer yes or no?"* Take action.

Making good decisions will build your confidence. Using a positive thinking mindset will help you develop a plan to make good decisions. Here's an example of using a plan to help make a good decision.

Let' suppose:

For years you have been driving along the same route from home to work and back home everyday for the past 10 years. Then, one day you discover there may be a shorter route with less traffic. So you methodically determine the benefits of using the shorter route. You analyze the good and the bad, the pros and the cons of making the route change.

- Are the roads on the alternate route safe from dangerous activity?
- Are the roads in good condition?
- Do you have to go through neighborhoods that have school zones with school bus stops?
- Does the new route offer a scenic view vs. an industrial view? Which would be your pleasure?

Although this is an easy and simple example in decision making, this outlines the type of process a positive thinking mind uses in helping to make good decisions.

A positive mindset says that every decision we make has consequences from the smallest degree of importance. Once you obtain a track record proving a history of making good decisions your confidence levels will sometimes appear off the charts. And it is a good thing to have super confidence moving forward into your future.

Confidence builds a solid character that makes good decisions. And making good decisions builds your confidence.

HEALTHY BODY healthy mind makes good decisions

When we earnestly work on improving ourselves with exercise and a healthy foods diet we will automatically experience a natural self-satisfying confidence. This is our positive energy DNA saluting our efforts.

Create your customized timetable for eating, exercising and sleeping. Once you have started a diet and exercise routine it will be easier to adjust your lifestyle of work and play into the routine. Then tweak your routine as you go along.

It has been my experience that the hardest part to every journey towards self-improvement is to commit to a start date. Don't haggle with yourself. Pick a date and get started. Make a sincere commitment to yourself. And once you commit don't quit. Daily, remind yourself that you are training your body and mind for your lifetime. And while you are working on keeping your body in good physical health your positive thinking mind is continuously sending up to date progress alerts to your subconscious. This is an auto-response internal notification process written into your DNA. And it is designed to keep you mentally focused on your positive thinking plans and goals. It is a constant reminder that you are using your positive thinking mindset.

The confidence builder of positive thinking

To build your confidence continue to do the following:

- Keep setting goals.
- Keep accomplishing goals.
- Keep having successes
- Keep celebrating your successes.

A positive thinking mindset stays motivated. And remains positive by doing positive works. Everyday remind yourself to stay constantly aware of your immediate surroundings by always keeping in touch with your natural senses of sight, sound and touch.

- Exercise your eyes. Throughout the day focus your eyes on distance and close up views. Do a panoramic scan of your surrounding views. Rotate your pupils 360 degrees. This exercise resets your visual focus.
- Utilize deep breathing exercises throughout the day. Breathe in through your nose and breathe out through your mouth counting 1,2,3…
- Actually 'smell the coffee,' which means activate your 'nosey' sense of smell, regularly. Sniff fresh air!
- Touchy-feely the soft pedals of a rose; or baby's face. Remind yourself of the sensations of touch.
- Give a hug! Experience the transfer of human warmth daily! Hug a body. Hug your pet!
- Listen for the sounds of the morning birds singing, rushing waters, blowing winds.
- As often as you can visit the sun rising or setting.
- (Here, add your own ideas of getting in touch with your senses). Do it!

Consistently refocus your senses for optimum experiences of awareness. Additionally, stay aware of your inner spirit connections. We are spirit beings and we are connected to all of Nature. We share similar DNA molecules. Our building blocks are related by creation.

- the birds, the bees
- the trees
- the animals
- the wind and seas
- the mountains and the plains

Being positive is using self visualization with self talk affirmations that help to keep you motivated to do the actions that produce positive works such as:

- Helping a neighbor or stranger without looking for repayment.
- Making yourself available for someone in need who has less than you.
- Sharing with others your God given skills or talents without reservation or payment.

Having confidence in your positive thinking is a learned state of mind that anyone can achieve with a true desire to be and think positive.

POSITIVE AFFIRMATIONS BUILD confidence

What are affirmations? The definition of affirmation is something declared to be true; a positive statement or judgement. When you intentionally and purposely desire to create and develop a positive thinking mindset you are self-improving your lifestyle for the better.

Repeating positive affirmations throughout your day can change the process of thinking negative thoughts. When you use positive affirmations daily, you are making yourself mentally more aware of the thoughts you are thinking. Affirmations are word phrases you create to be repeated to yourself to help change your thinking attitude and behavior. This process is most effective when you use honest word phrases about yourself with a sincere desire to change how you think about yourself.

Do the work of writing down on paper all of positive thoughts you have about yourself. Make the effort to create a daily routine of saying your affirmations out loud visualizing them in your mind. It is recommended to recite your affirmations in front of a mirror to help visualize that it is you making the requests. From your heart with deep and sincere devotion, repeat phrases like these.

- I am a strong person.
- I conquer my goals one by one.
- I get things done

These are examples to get you started. But do create your own word phrases that identify exactly what it is you want to achieve. Practice reciting your affirmations in the morning when you wake up, while getting dressed, at work and throughout the day. Here are a few more examples.

- I am honest.
- I am a good person.
- I love everybody.
- Every day I get better.
- I will reach my goals.
- I do not fail.
- I am success.

Allow affirmations to become part of your new lifestyle. Your powers of positive thinking that is already in your DNA is awakened when you recite your affirmations. Over time you will accomplish all of your goals using positive affirmations.

The power of saying "I'm sorry"

"I'm sorry. Please accept my apologies."

"I apologize. I am so sorry."

Repeatedly using the phrase *"I'm sorry"* will never build confidence. It is character defeating to constantly use the statement, *"I'm sorry."* There is a phrase from the movie Forest Gump: *"Stupid is as stupid does."* Likewise, "Sorry is like sorry does."

Sorry is a feeling of regret or penitence that draws on the soul when used correctly. The true value to feeling sorry is to have empathy from your soul for another human being; to actually feel hurt or anguish for someone, to share in their pain of an issue, problem or loss.

But when we so quickly offer an apology and say "I'm sorry" what does it really mean and what message are we trying to send to the person to whom we are offering the apology?

When a customer makes a telephone call to a company to register a complaint or to inquire of a product or service the receptionists almost always immediately apologizes for any and all problems the company may have caused the customer. And the apology is extended to any personal discomfort the customer may have at that moment while on the telephone. The receptionists continues to apologize for the slightest inconvenience the customer may have. Even to the point of apologizing for future unforeseen events!

Is it necessary to apologize for someone else's error? Is an apology required from someone other than the person that created the problem? I don't think so. Offering a needless apology is a demeaning act for the person making the apology. It draws on and depletes the integrity of their character. In a needless apology why should someone 'feel sorry' for something they did not do?

In all of life we are never responsible for someone else's mistake. And as such we are not obligated to apologize. It is imperative that whoever caused the problem should be the one to apologize for the problem: If a sincere apology is actually needed.

Positive thinking says that apologizing for someone's mistake is wasted energy. You are depleting your 'soul' whenever you give a sincere apology for someone else's mistake.

Positive thinkers don't manufacture or create apologies for problems they did not create. This way they are assured to keep their positive mental attitude in good working order to withstand their own problems and mistakes when a sincere apology is truly needed.

The company receptionists who apologizes countless times throughout their workday have unknowingly weakened their character with mental fatigue. They have bared their souls throughout the day apologizing repeatedly for everyone else's mistakes. At the end of the day they go to their homes exhausted and drained of their character only to return tomorrow for more of the same. By the end of a busy week they are beat down and mentally tired trying to figure out why they have so little energy left in their souls to share with their family of loved ones.

Use your innate DNA powers of positive thinking to tell your mind to stop making unnecessary apologies. There is no reason to say, "I'm sorry," for matters you have no influence or control of. We all make mistakes and at times when our actions are wrong a sincere apology is needed. *"I apologize,"* or *"I empathize,"* are the optimum expressions to be used in these real situations. The use of the words, "I am sorry," may imply a failure and indicate some amount of responsibility for the negative outcome of the situation which you may not be responsible for.

This argument may seem minor in detail and substance but it is major in personal character development. Avoid this negative. You will limit your powers of positive thinking if you are constantly apologizing. Especially for things you had no involvement in or control of. Also, in most instances the apology you are expressing probably has no sincere impact on the person you are delivering the apology to. Most likely they have already anticipated the apology forthcoming because it is considered the polite and proper norm of society to do so. The apology is now given by the 'giver' without sincere empathy and expected by the receiver without sincere appreciation.

When we appropriately own up to our own mistakes we can only hope it is enough and equal to the challenge of being responsible for our own misgivings to say, "I am sorry."

Save your apologies for your mistakes. Take responsibility for your actions only. Stop apologizing for someone else. Allow them to pay their own debt. If your intent is to express empathy to the person for the situation, kindly respond, *"I empathize with you for the problem that has been created."* And leave it there.

Let's all stop apologizing for negative situations we did not create or have any influence in their creation. I'm sorry can be a powerful statement to convey the sincerity of any message. Don't use this statement if it is not needed and sincerely meant. It has true power coming from a truly sincere person. My suggestion for these moments is to save all your empathy and sympathy for real lamenting situations where emotions are truly needed.

The takeaway here is don't waste your positive energy and positive attitude on useless actions that reduce your positive thinking mindset. Apologizing for actions you have no control over is pure wasted energy and reduces your confidence levels.

ALTERNATIVES TO MAKING needless apologies

Consider these responses in situations where you would usually say "I'm sorry."

- I understand. So let me help you.
- No worries. I can help you with this.
- We will do better next time.
- Let's see how I can help
- Okay. I got this for you.
- Let me work on it.
- Well, let me show you how it should be done.
- I empathize with you. Let me see how I can help.

Did you notice that all these alternative responses are POSITIVE?

Forgot making unnecessary insincere apologies. In most instances of apology the person you are apologizing to quickly forgets and doesn't retain any memory of the apology. In essence the I'm sorry apology has become a ceremonial conversation piece that is discarded as fast as it is presented. No one remembers. But your soul does. Stop needless apologies.

REFLECTIONS ON TODAY - confidence for tomorrow

It's the end of the day. Time for bed.

But this night, stop and take a moment to reflect on the day.

In your mind review your days' activities.

Did you get caught up in some type of disagreements? Bar brawl? Road Rage?? An argument at the office? The kids?

But now it's bedtime. Mentally unwind. Review the days activities in your mind.

Search for conversations or events of the day where opportunities to learn something were present. Make note of the fact that you were either aware of the opportunity or that you missed the opportunity.

Note also that a missed opportunity can reappear to give you a second chance. Be vigilant.

Now, take out the trash. Visualize, in your mind the act of throwing out the negative things of your day into the trash bin. Throw out all the things negative that you don't need to remember. This is where the trash goes.

What is important is the fact that you are now 'keeping score' by recalling the events of your day. You are creating a mental process that will help you to think about your day; each day looking for clues in your daily thinking.

Remind yourself everyday to be completely focused and aware of all situations that require your attention.

- Be aware of the people you interact with on a regular basis such as your co-workers, family and friends. Know who they are. Who's a positive person? Who is a negative person?
- Remove all discouraging and disparaging words and remarks from your vocabulary.
- Avoid using profanity because this allows you to accept more profanity into your life. Practice the realization that profanity is on the extreme side of the spectrum and there is no reason to behave in an extreme manor at anytime.
- Rationalize your thinking and speaking habits to be pleasant, appealing and acceptable to all people.
- Make conscious decisions as to when to speak and when to be silent. Avoid speaking all the time in conversations. Intentionally allow the other person equal talk time. Practice listening more.
- In relationships visualize only the good. If there is something you don't like, you don't have to mention it just

because it is there. If it is preventing you from being positive in the relationship or it is something that may be detrimental to the relationship going forward then it needs to be addressed. Otherwise, let it be.

And at all costs avoid getting 'Stuck on Stupid'. It can make you,'Dumber than Dirt!' 'Stuck on Stupid' and 'Dumber than Dirt' are expressions I think of when I perceive someone who '*Doesn't see the forest, for the trees.*'

To explain. Our forests contains all sorts of goodies and treasures of nature. When we take the time to examine what is in our forests (the mind) we find a treasure trove of beneficial items for our life. But for some people they find a tree, one tree (one issue) that seems to satisfy them and they never move from that one tree. They are genuinely stuck in their own mind on that one tree and cannot see the beauty or value of all the other trees that make up the forest. They can't see the entire forest (life) because of that one tree (issue). And subsequently they become stuck and that makes it stupid. They mentally agree to see only what they want to see; the one tree. They're stuck...on stupid. And to be stuck on stupid for any extended period of time will result in being 'dumber than dirt.'

Everyday, using the confidence in our abilities to improve our thinking processes, we learn to make better decisions that will improve the quality of our lives.

CHAPTER 3 RECAP

Good Decisions Build Confidence

- It's all in your mind
- Negative thoughts are like bullies

- Find confidence in your decision making
- Healthy body healthy mind makes good decisions
- The confidence builder of positive thinking
- Positive affirmations build confidence
- The power of saying "I'm sorry"
- Alternatives to making needless apologies
- Reflections on today - confidence for tomorrow

MAKE REAL ACCOMPLISHMENTS

Use your positive mind

Achievements are the goals we aim to reach within a designed plan of action. As you successfully achieve each goal within the plan, these items become accomplishments. Every achievement accomplished within the plan deserves recognition by celebration. A celebration of each achievement within the plan is recognition of your accomplishment: You did it!

Most times when it's a small achievement, a slight wink and a nod to yourself mentally is adequate. But understand it must be mandatory in your thinking mind to recognize the slightest upward movement you make in your plan. For a more distinctive show of appreciation for your larger achievements make the celebration a bit more noticeable to yourself with a lunch or dinner date.

Here is an example of when to celebrate the successes of your achievements within your plan.

A typical problem we all may have had at some point in our lives is staying up late into the night when we know we should get to bed early to be better prepared for tomorrow. The results of staying up late is that you are not getting enough sleep. And throughout the next day you are feeling tired and sleepy. It's time to set a goal to get more sufficient sleep at night to have more energy throughout the day.

The plan is to create a scheduled routine to get to bed early to ensure sufficient sleep time. And you want to accomplish this goal in 30 days. First step is to write out a scheduled routine for tomorrow's activities that includes the following:

1. Make a schedule for the next day activities. (repeat every night)

2. Set a specific time to get to bed early.

3. Get up each morning at the same time.

4. Start your scheduled activities for the day.

After 10 days have passed and you have maintained your plan instructions for each step in the plan, 1, 2, 3 and 4, it is time to celebrate yourself mentally with a wink and a nod. This is an acknowledgment to yourself that you are on the right path doing the right thing to reach your planned goal. Repeat this acknowledgement at the next 10 day interval. At the end of the 30 days, as set by your plan, you will have achieved success. Now it is reward time and you should go out for a full lunch or dinner celebration with family or friends to acknowledge your accomplishment: reaching your goal. Always celebrate your achievements no matter how small. This act of self celebrating is encouraging and helps to breed self-confidence. For long term confidence and success make it a permanent part of your planning to always celebrate each achievement. The mental celebrations of the little steps along the way are the building blocks that help reinforce your beliefs that your positive thinking mindset is working, just as you planned. This is a very important and meaningful part of your overall planning for life long success. The acknowledgement celebrations remind you that your persistence paid off and to 'keep your eye on the prize.' Commit to completing each element of your plan using the step by step; 1, 2, 3 procedure.

MAKE plans to be positive

Use these affirmations as a part of your plan to help you get started. Over time, modify or replace them with your own affirmation statements.

- I am a positive thinking person. I get things done.
- I am positive because I was born positive.
- I am a part of the universe of positive creations.
- Positive thinking is in my DNA.
- Positive thinking works for me all the time.

Be consistent. Have a scheduled routine to follow. Using a set routine for everyday creates discipline. Sticking to your plan, look forward to reaching your goals in the order you set for scheduled achievements by remaining consistent.

Set your plan with strict attention to breaking down the time slots into half hours. Then set the half hours into 15 minute intervals. Schedule your time in small manageable time slots until you can become more comfortable with the bigger time intervals. For example:

Wake up and start your day.

- 15 -20 in the bathroom to get ready for the day.

- 10-15 for a light breakfast only.
- 10-20 minutes planning the day/meditations
- 10-15 to get dressed
- 20-30 drive/commute to work

In scheduling, set your focus on achieving one task at a time. No multi-tasking. In the beginning multi-tasking will only crowd your thinking thoughts. Once you reach a certain level of achieving your objectives multi-tasking can then become a choice. But to get started focus your scheduling on one task at a time.

As you are moving forward working your plan you will begin to notice that your mind starting to percolate all sorts of ideas coming from your newly formed thought patterns. Take advantage of the benefits these new ideas are bringing. Keep writing materials or voice recording material available and close at hand. Good thoughts come fast and unexpectedly. And they will leave just as quickly. So keep pen and paper nearby at all times to keep track of your new positive thinking thoughts and ideas.

You are now encouraging your mind to be observant of its thinking processes. All random thinking which the mind does all the time will now be noted by your conscious mind. At this point you are completely aware of your thinking thoughts. It is now, time to direct your mind to think the thoughts you want it to think. When we are intentionally focused on our thinking patterns we become capable of labeling and identifying when and what we are actually thinking. This is your positive energy DNA being reflected onto your conscious mental thinking.

Be realistic and disciplined to control your telephone calls and internet activities. Create a schedule of certain times within the day that you handle emails and internet activities. Avoid making unnecessary immediate responses to emails and telephone calls. These are the distractions that can take you off schedule completely changing your positive thinking patterns.

Include meditations, routine exercises, affirmations/prayer into your schedule at a minimum 3 times per week at first. Later on you may want to add more items to your everyday routine.

A perfect time for meditation and relaxation would be to take one entire day out of the week and do no work. Use this time to release the pressures of working your regular job and working on your positive mindset schedule. Take a break. And notice the rush of ideas that come to you when you are fully relaxed and at peace within yourself. Working your plan of action with moments of peace and relaxation will allow your success to be therapeutic.

There are huge benefits in successful planning. The biggest benefit is the successful accomplishment of the plan. Follow your plan step by step, 1,2,3.

Create your first plan to get started. Conquer it and create another plan to accomplish your next set of goals.

To have a positive thinking mindset for your life where you make real accomplishments, be sure to add these three main objectives to your everyday lifestyle.

1. *"Improve your health. Watch what you eat."*

- Start eating healthy foods only!
- Drink plenty of water as part of your overall diet.
- Stop eating fatty foods and processed foods.
- No more midnight snacking.
- Reduce your intake of all alcoholic beverages.
- No more binge drinking at all.
- No smoking.
- No tobacco products

- No vaping
- No cannabis products (unless medically prescribed)
- According to your age get the right amount of sleep every night

2. *"Improve your physical body. Exercise regularly."*

- Get into a routine of making physical movement of your body. Simply take a walk! Our muscles become aged and dysfunctional when we refuse to exercise them. Muscle memory does not age. As long as you work the muscles they will respond no matter the age. If it is hard for you to get into an exercise routine all at once, pace yourself and develop a schedule according to your honesty with yourself. Don't force it. If one day a week works fine in the beginning, then go with it knowing that you will need to add more exercise time in the future.
- Be kind and lenient with yourself. Most important to remember is that you are in control and this is your body, your time and you make or break the rules as you see fit.
- Know to yourself that if you stop YOU CAN START AGAIN. It's ok.
- If doing exercises is not what you desire accept this as a fact about yourself. But know that a healthy mind with a healthy body is necessary for an optimum positive thinking mindset.
- And remember a daily walk does count as daily exercise.

3. *"Improve your thinking mind. Read."*

- Read more to create more positive thinking thoughts. Reading is fundamental to learning. Use your positive thinking energy to bring the positive thoughts forward that will encourage you to read more.

- Prayer, meditation and affirmations are the best techniques for improving the thinking mind. In the privacy of your home in front of a mirror recite out loud the affirmation statements you have chosen for your purposes. Throughout your day mentally repeat your affirmations everywhere you go. After your very first time doing this routine pay attention to your thoughts. Look for a difference in your thinking patterns.

In a private space practice remaining physically still and being quiet. Do this everyday for 10 minutes. This exercise allows your mind to establish peace with your body and soul. Be consistent here. Your mental attitude means everything to making a successful long lasting positive mindset change.

Thinking with a positive mindset also helps in the following ways.

- Brings peace to your soul.
- Calms your overall attitude.
- Helps in negotiating and settling negative issues with others.
- Eliminates the need to worry.
- Causes a significant reduction in negative overthinking.

In time you will learn that the majority of your worrisome and troubling issues are much easier to resolve than you had previously thought. Everyday physically practice emptying your mind of useless habits you know you need to get rid of: Such as staying up late at night when you know you need to get to bed earlier.

Allow the powers of positive affirmations to tell you to expect good things to come your way when you eliminate a bad habit. Make a solemn promise to yourself to purposely avoid using all negative words of profane and negative talk. Avoid all negative activity with the people you interact with on a regular basis. This pertains especially to those who are closest to you.

Refrain from holding a grudge against anyone. Holding on to a grudge will certainly interrupt your progress. Grudges are stumbling blocks on your road to a positive thinking mindset for life.

Make friends with positive thinking people. You will have more interesting life fulfilling discussions with positive thinking people because of their natural positivity.

Find out who you can really trust in your circle of influence of family and friends. Identify the personalities within your family and friends as to who is positive and who is negative. Immediately end all relationships with known liars, cheaters and deceivers. In my personal experiences I have found family and friends to be the most apparent sources of negative energy. They can be very detrimental to your progress if you continue to cater to the negativity of their whims and wishes. Remember, they don't know what you know about positive thinking energy.

But remain confident that you will find positive ways to work around their negativity as opposed to choosing to eliminating them from your circle of influence altogether. It will be much better for you and for them if you can stand out from the crowd as a true example of someone who is living with a positive thinking attitude.

Rely on your positive thinking

Make these all important elements a part of your strategy in developing your positive thinking mind.

Awareness. Being aware is simply paying attention to your surroundings. Make solid concentrated efforts to physically look at everything around you. This routine helps to keep you mentally focused and alert at all times. Awareness is the first mental function of our thinking mind.* When we use this function to its fullest capacity we are on a mental alert focusing, absorbing and processing all the visual data of our immediate surroundings. We are paying strict attention.

Acceptance. Wherever you are currently in life, fully accept your position.

Mark this time as a solid beginning point to changing your lifestyle. You are establishing a 'Point A'. Do the work needed to move on to Point B etc. Step by step, 1,2,3.

Focus. Constantly remind yourself to stay focused on the objectives necessary to reach your goals. You will always be presented with distractions. Be strong and stay focused.

Fear. Have no fear of losing. If you begin and then stop, don't give up and accept defeat. Pick up and start again. Maintain the mental position: *"I am in charge. I make the rules about my life."* On this journey you set up the rules. Once you begin know that you are using a positive thinking mindset to succeed and you have set your mind to 'finish.' Have no fear of failure.

Throughout your journey at any time along the way if you need a pause or a pause happens outside of your control, know that it is 'ok' because you are in charge and you have the power to reset the rules to begin again. Stay committed knowing that what you have started you will finish.

---

* See Resources - from the book Overthinking? 7 Steps to Finding Peace from Overthinking Stress Anxiety and Worry

Accomplish your goals

Use diligent work efforts to achieve your goals everyday. When you make the achievements in your plan to reach your goals you are on the right track to achieve success.

You are doing the right things at the right time for all the right reasons if you are using these guidelines.

- Set realistic goals. Goals that are reachable within your lifestyle and within your abilities to achieve them.
- Make preparations to learn more about your topic/subject matter. Read more about your topics of interests.
- Stay motivated to succeed. Have discussions on your topics of interest with family, friends and associates. But only with those you trust.
- Remind yourself of your goals by listening to yourself talk when you are reciting your affirmations.
- Be resourceful. Reach out and find a mentor or a knowledgeable partner to help qualify your ideas.
- Stay Persistent always working on your plan. 'Tweak' your plan regularly to keep it up to date within your goals.
- Remain consistently focused on 'your prize' to succeed.
- Maintain a healthy diet with an exercise routine. You want to enjoy the benefits of a healthy mind and body when you reach your goals.
- Look forward to celebration time!

PLAN TO SUCCEED and never give up

As I stated earlier, *"The hardest part of any project is to get started."*

Commit to begin. Have a positive mindset that says once you start the project the project will end. Be committed to never give up, never give in, never give out.

Don't have any fear of failing to complete the project once you have started. Constantly remind yourself that this is your self appointed project and you make or break the rules as you see necessary to complete the project. And if you don't complete the project within the time period you wanted don't become discouraged. You just may need time to relax. So take some time off, away from the project. It's ok to set a new finish/completion date.

Procrastination does not mean the end. You can always pick up and start again. Never give up on your ideas and desires. As long as you are alive you can start again with a new plan to win.

Never give in to failure or quitting. Re adjusting the plan to suit your needs is part of the overall planned design to succeed for your life. It's your plan and you make all the decisions to accomplish your goals.

The power of desire

A major key ingredient to acquiring the knowledge needed to think positive on a consistent basis is desire. Without this main component you will not achieve positive thinking everyday. You must earnestly desire to be positive. Why? Because this is where your true source of power exists: in your soul of desires. If you truly want to live a positive thinking lifestyle know that you can have it because the positive energy is already inside of you: in your DNA.

But you must earnestly desire to think positive. A positive person desires to be a positive thinker at all times. A positive person earnestly desires to avoid all negative concepts and positions. When you seriously desire to think positive and believe you can be a positive person you begin to think like someone who will one day rule 'his/her' world. This is the positive thinking mindset. Acquiring and thinking with a positive mindset is literally:

- planning ahead to be positive in all areas of your life;
- getting ready and being prepared mentally for whatever life situation may come your way.

Each day of your life can be a new beginning, a true new birth. And each new awakening day brings possibilities of something great and exciting for you when you think of having a positive lifestyle.

Aspire and desire to be positive and you will be positive. Wake up each day and get your new beginnings going.

Get better every year with planned optimism

Use your positive power of thought and declare to yourself that you will make improvements in your life to get better every year. Set a favorite or significant date (such as anniversary dates because they are easier to remember) to mark the beginning of a new journey to accomplish a constructive life change. Or, let each New Year's Day be your natural marker.

I share this true story with you about one of my life changing accomplishments.

For several years living in Connecticut, I operated my own real estate brokerage, America's Homes & Communities Real Estate. One night I went out for the evening to one of my favorite restaurants located in the downtown business district. Many times after a real estate closing I would meet friends and associates for celebratory dinners with drinks and sometimes dancing. The managers and the staff at this particular restaurant were always cordial to all of its customers. The establishment maintained a 5 star reputation for its food and atmosphere for many years.

Approaching the New Year I went to the restaurant to schedule a party for friends. While waiting for the hostess I noticed a business buddy who was eyeing me from across the room. His eyes met mine and he gestured coming over to meet me.

"Bryanscott? Is that you? Man! You look great! You are one of the few people who I have ever known who seem to get better and better year after year!" He said it again, "You look great!" Naturally I accepted his compliment graciously with sincere respect for his kind words. And later when I returned home the words of his compliment came to me again.

I looked into the mirror and would easily agree with what he had said. I had noticeably changed from last year! And then I remembered. It was in my plans of two years past to make significant changes in my thinking. My planned determination at that time was to get mentally focused on improving my mental health and physical well-being. And it was all because I had suffered a major setback that year; a devastating real estate loss. A shopping center development that I was working on had fallen apart at the final preposed closing date. I was to be a principal partner in a 70k+ shopping plaza. My financial and business interests were:

- a 20% part owner of the plaza;
- liquor store owner and tenant;
- the property leasing manger for the entire shopping plaza.

My company, AHC Real Estate had worked for a little more than a year and a half, non-stop on this project. I coordinated the land acquisition proposals, site designs and state and local approvals. The bank financing was handled by the developer. All of my hard work on this project ended after three postponed property/land acquisition closings. On the day of the last preposed closing the bank that was supplying the funds to close, filed for bankruptcy: on that day. No shopping plaza for Bryanscott.

I nestled into a 'poor Bryanscott pity me' lifestyle for about 4 months. And then it happened. I woke one morning and made the decision to get back to reality. I admitted I lost; It was over. Accepting defeat I challenged myself to change my thinking mindset to subsequently change my lifestyle. Having a new positive thinking mindset became my goal. I told myself, *"Forget about the past. Let's move on."*

It was about two years ago that I had made the decision to actually think more clearly about life and make the necessary positive changes. Determined, I accepted the past and moved on to begin my comeback. Wherever possible I instituted positive thinking ideas and attitudes toward everything I did. From my readings of Dr. Wayne Dyer on being positive, I learned that if I sincerely wanted to change my life I would have to adopt a daily routine with a new way of thinking about myself. Based on what I was learning this is how I began to make the needed changes in my life.

- Physically, I started exercising everyday. Once in a while I would skip a day or two. But I was committed to winning so whenever I got lazy I simply regrouped my thoughts and returned to my exercise routine.
- Changed my diet and began eating salads, vegetables and fruits.
- Reduce red meat intake to once a month or not at all. I replaced red meats with chicken or fish.
- Reduced my alcohol intake by canceling out all hard liquors, first. Resigned to having just a beer or two, or a glass of wine for celebrations.

- Stopped partying so hard. No more late hours 'clubbing and socializing' at the bars.
- Dedicated one day a week for serious non-work activities and simply relaxed listening to soft music and taking walks in the park. Or go for a drive down by the shore.
- And for the main event I committed to made it a habit to read the New King James Version of the Bible everyday.
- In Jesus name I would pray every night.

Optimism with confidence will grow when you're working your plan. Everyday use the positive affirmations you have created. They help to remind you to stay committed. Affirmations can be your triggers to keep you motivated to succeed.

With optimism and a plan you will make real accomplishments. And get better every year.

"Hey Bryanscott... You look great!"

CHAPTER 4 RECAP

Make Real Accomplishments

- Use your positive mind
- Make plans to be positive
- Rely on your positive thinking
- Accomplish your goals
- Plan to succeed and never give up!
- The power of desire
- Get better every year with planned optimism (ACTUAL EVENT)

ENJOY LOVE & PEACE WITH FAMILY & OTHERS

The positive attitude is love

To receive real love is to be available to give real love.

Be willing to give of yourself first so that the other person can actually see that you truly have love for them.

But love has nothing to do with mental acuity. You don't have to be smart to be loved or to give love. Love is a lining, like a sheet or blanket, placed into everything of nature. The beasts of the fields and the creatures of the deep seas need love and share love with one another. Love is universally foundational. It is easily identifiable and found in every living thing.

Love has always been a part of you from your beginning. Speak to the love inside of you more often. Give some love; share a hug. And watch your personal love attraction levels grow!

Sharing your love and peace with family and friends creates environments where everyone can feel safe and wanted. Allow your positive energy to grow and flow with the power to encourage all in the family to behave in the same sharing and caring spirit. Don't hesitate to show them just how much you love them with your actions of affection; a kiss, a hug, a few kind words. Show them by your example just how beneficial it is for everyone to have open communications sharing their feelings in honesty and respect without judgement of one another. Put your positive attitude on display for them to see that your way of thinking is to live and let live in peace and harmony. Emphasize this each day because each day brings new challenges with more needs for more love.

When loved ones are expressing their sincere feelings, listen to them with an attentive ear as 'to hear a pin drop.' You may not give them the answers they want to hear but your listening attention is priceless to in their eyes.

Share your love for the family by showing respect for their unique personalities. Let them know that in your decision making processes their opinions are taken seriously at all times. Additionally;

- Always offer your support;
- Share your quality time with them;
- Accept and respect their unique differences;
- Express your gratitude for their love and support of you.

The familial sense of love and peace is not easy to gain and nor is it guaranteed to last. The strength of your positive attitude is required at all times to help maintain a strong family unit that enjoys love and peace for everyone.

Being understanding, compassionate and willing to forgive with persistent patience must be openly demonstrated by the elders and leaders of the family. And each member of the family must be supportive of one another especially at times of troubles and pain.

This timely support is very much needed to prevent anyone from feeling alone, left out and forgotten.

Routinely show your concerns for the safety and well being of each family member so that there is no ambiguity or question as to what are your sincere concerns for all in the family. Share with them your positive attitude towards forgiveness by letting go of past indiscretions and wrongdoings. Show them by your actions that you carry no grudges or ill will against anyone: family, friend or foe. Be sure to share plenty of "Give me a hug" moments for everyone.

Include setting clear and certain boundaries that are designed to maintain the health and well-being of all in the family. No profane or ill moral conduit can be accepted. Negative behaviors must be identified and chastised immediately before they have a chance to become something harmful. Family counseling may be needed and if so don't hesitate to contact someone for support. Use your positive thinking mindset to identify and resolve issues before they can become problems.

If you are the one who is counted on to produce a healthy environment for the family to live and grow in, don't be afraid to step up to the plate and give it your very best. Remember other family leaders succeed and you are capable of succeeding as well.

Positive people avoid negative people

For the routine maintenance of your everyday positive thinking mindset do your best to avoid negative people. It is said 'in nature' opposites attract. And negative people are attracted to positive thinking people. When a positive thinking person accepts a long term relationship with a negative person the positive person will loose part of their positive thinking energy. Avoid the negative because they will become a drain on your positive thinking energies.

Here is a list of negative personalities the positive thinking person avoids.

- Alcohol abusers
- Liars - Deceivers
- Thieves -Shoplifters
- Whisperers
- Grifters - Those who use and live off others
- Womanizers - Masochists
- Drug dealers and drug users
- Pedophiles -molesters
- Narcissists
- Sex addicts
- Pornography addicts
- Impersonators - Con artist
- Toxic persons - gaslighters

And this is the short list! All of these personalities have a social mood disorder or illness that is most likely complicated with severe overthinking issues brought on with cognitive distortions. Long term association with them will literally stop you from ever achieving your goals of having a positive thinking mindset. Their negative attitudes will block your naturally positive thinking powers.

Know that negative minded people will absorb your positive energy and leave you with nothing of value; only memories of a weak relationship.

Generally speaking, most negative minded people are scantly aware of their negative thinking patterns. It's their lifestyle, their ways of living they have allowed them to be vulnerable to the negative influences in their life. And now they don't know how to live any other way.

You will lose yourself and your time of life if you continue to associate with negative thinking people. They may require professional help. Direct them to the professionals who are in the business of helping people who suffer with negative personality disorders. Let them know without any hesitation that you do not have the power to help them change their negative thinking personalities.

There are also certain events and gatherings where the positive thinking person should avoid. Whenever you are aware of an event or an occasion where there exists a high probability of some type of negative activity can occur, do your best to avoid the event. Give value to your time and don't waste it on a known negative atmosphere.

Here are a few circumstances where you should prepare for the possibility of negative behavior.

- When driving in traffic always be prepared to avoid road rage attacks.
- Having a disagreement with a store clerk or salesperson. Call for the manager. But remain calm.
- At a family gathering that can easily produce arguments. Avoid debates, especially if alcohol is being served. No need to raise your blood pressure levels talking about issues you have no influence or control over.

We all have had past situations where we believe we could have done something different to have created a better outcome. Use this bit of wisdom: "An once of prevention is always better than a pound of cure." It is positive thinking to avoid a negative situation.

Time is the commodity of life

Our lives are everything within time. No time, no life. Time is the most valuable resource of your life. Live the times of your life prudently. Avoid wasting your time of life thinking of matters that contain not one scintilla of beneficial knowledge to improve your everyday enjoyment of life.

Appreciate your time. Be wise to use your time for quality moments. Look to get the greatest value out of living life.

Time is fleeting, going fast, never to return. How you use the time in your life is exactly how you will enjoy your living.

Everyone desires to be happy and safe and this is what we work towards; to be happy, contented and safe each day of our existence. This is a never-ending chore until the day we die.

Each day is a new day with new and different challenges co-mingled with the old challenges of yesterday. And in all reality this is exactly how we spend our journey of life; overcoming the daily challenges in our lives. Subconsciously what we all strive for is to have a better everyday life, one day at a time.

Enjoy your life one day at a time

Life actually exists only one day at a time. And the true apex of living life comes from the joys of being alive, each day. Every morning as we open our eyes a new day is dawning, a new life is born. Be thankful that you have received this morning; the gift of life for another day.

Be nice to yourself. Do not demand perfection from your works. Don't be so hard on yourself when you make a mistake. And it is important that you forgive yourself and move on from any and all mistakes you have made. Remind yourself,

"I have another day."

Apply this rule throughout your lifetime: Allow nothing and no one to be more important than you and your life. The only exception to this rule is the love you have for your Creator. Because of Him you are allowed another chance at life for another day: one day at a time.

Additionally, get mentally focused on being genuinely kind to everyone you meet. Yes. Everyone! Create a mental platform where you can stay focused on sharing your kindness with others on a regular basis: Like everyday!

Greet someone new with a sincere smile that says you're happy to see them. Know that each time you share a little bit of kindness with someone your positive thinking energy gets stimulated. Eagerly volunteer your time and energy to share yourself with family and friends. Volunteering is refreshing to the soul and very rewarding to the spirit.

Practice keeping company with positive people who genuinely show respect and admiration for you, your ideas and your life principles.

The benefits of a daily hug

A stranger, who is now a friend offered to give me a hug when we first met! She shared with me some of the scientifically explained benefits of hugging. And after we hugged I actually experienced a comforting feeling throughout the rest of the day mentally and physically, just from her one 20 second hug.

Sharing our feelings with others is a universal needy human condition: We all need one another. And we can easily communicate these feelings when we intentionally extend ourselves. Offer a hug. When you give a hug you are also getting a hug. It is said that a sincere hug of 20 seconds or more has a therapeutic effect on the body and mind. This warm embrace produces the hormone called oxytocin, a stress reducing hormone written into our DNA.

Consider getting into a habit of offering sincere hugs to family and friends throughout your everyday. Medical studies have shown that hugging gives the following benefits:

- Stimulates the thymus gland
- Encourages self-esteem
- Stimulates oxytocin
- Helps to develop an attitude of patience
- Reduces stress
- Relive needless worry
- Calm anxiety
- Release pleasure hormone dopamine
- Activates Serotonin levels[*]

The positive energy of a simple hug is also transmitted to our pets. You can see just how warmed and excited they respond to you when you give them a hug. Positive energy is in their DNA.

Now after I had learned about the power of the hug I eagerly offered a hug to my neighbor Christine. She agreed and opened her arms. I extended myself and gently wrapped my arms around her. I held her in my grasp for the 20 seconds. When I released her she exclaimed " Well. That was a bit much." I replied " The oxytocin kicked in." " It was more than oxytocin," she quipped.

---

[*]   See Resources - 10 Health Benefits of Hugging, backed by Science

Offer a surprise hug to someone with the hope of generating a pay-it-forward hugging marathon. This is all positive action and a win-win situation for all who participate. Share with someone just how grateful you are for what good they may have done for you. Give them a hug!

Have genuine love for others

During a certain period in my life I held an Insurance Brokers License. During those times I was once hired by a small family owned insurance agency that specialized in all personal lines of insurance: Life Insurance, Auto Insurance, and Home Owners Insurance Protection.

When I first met Mr. Bradford the owner of the insurance agency I shared my credentials with him and he immediately offered me a probationary employment position as an in-office insurance policy writer. After working for just two months partially through the probationary employment period Mr. Bradford asked me if I would consider becoming an administrator as vice president with a possible percentage ownership of the company.

Having acquired a broker's licenses in all personal lines of insurance I had impressed Mr Bradford in such a short period of time with my employment history and work ethics.

I had worked for the large insurance companies, The Aetna and The Travelers Insurance Company as a pensions administrator for nearly 10 years. With college training in bookkeeping and accounting I coordinated the processes of posting to accounts and disbursing pension benefits to the employees of several large companies. Part of my duties required having on-going communications with the CFOs, CPAs and other pensions services administrators of their respective companies. My initial work history in the insurance industry started in individual life insurance policy sales where I did cold calling, door knocking and writing my own newspaper ads.

For Mr. Bradfords' company I used my skills and abilities and created the company's newspaper advertising and marketing materials. I redesigned the personal business cards and sales brochures for mailers and customer hand outs for meetings and seminars.

Mr. Bradford was an elder gentlemen who had been in the insurance business for much of his life and he felt the need to look forward to a retirement plan for the business he had made. He readily identified the potential I held for his desired purposes for his retirement. Once I had signed the agreement to become a principal in the company, Mr. Bradford contacted his sponsor company, Aetna Insurance and arranged the financing to pay my salary.

After four months of diligently working with Mr. Bradford, one Friday evening he called me at my home. I was just finishing up with dinner. Mr. Bradford called to asked me if I could 'pinch hit' for him by doing a health insurance seminar to a group of senior citizens the very next day, Saturday morning just before noon. I quickly replied that I would have no problem making such a presentation. But...I could not do this event for him tomorrow morning because I would need some time to prepare for it. He responded that there was no time to create a full blown presentation and he said that I should have enough knowledge to 'fluff' the presentation for the next morning.

I paused in my listening for a moment and thought of his idea of 'fluffing' through the seminar. I couldn't remember if I had ever 'fluffed' anything. I reasoned with myself that I probably could stumble through an hours' worth of 'fluff' to get through the presentation and this would please the boss. But then something positive came to my head. What if my fluff is a flop? What happens if I am asked a question I don't know the answer to but should know???

And then I got 'outside of my head' and hovered over my body to visualize my self thinking. I asked myself, "Am I having a 'cognitive distortion moment? Am I second guessing my abilities? Am I overthinking this situation?" No, I quickly rationalized and came to a decision. Mr. Bradford wanted me to perform in front of an audience to speak on healthcare benefits for seniors in approximately 12 hours. It was Friday night at 10 o'clock. To be properly prepared I must have at least 6 to 7 hours of sleep. Then I would need at least one and a half hours to comfortably refresh my knowledge of healthcare information to perform as accurately as possible without 'fluff.'

I returned to the telephone conversation and explained to Mr. Bradford; " I don't fluff. I know what I know and I will give you all I've got. But I don't fluff. I need a proper amount of time to prepare before making this type of presentation." Mr. Bradford quickly responded with one dismissively curt word; "Goodbye," as he hung up the telephone.

The following Monday morning I entered the office looking forward to asking Mr. Bradford how the seminar went. To my complete surprise my desk had been moved from the beautiful glass enclosure in the front of the office to a corner cubby hole next to the storage closet toward the rear exit door of the office. The secretary explained to me as I gazed in a state of sad bewilderment that Mr. Bradford had instructed her with a Sunday night telephone call to make the desk changes before I would arrive to the office that Monday morning.

The end result was that within the next few days Mr. Bradford and I agreed to cancel the employment arrangement and that I would leave his office immediately.

I felt as though I had lost a great opportunity for job growth and personal development that I was well suited for. But then I have also learned in life you can't loose something you don't really have.

My time with Mr. Brad ford was relatively short. I rationalize that Mr. Bradford was not offering me an honest opportunity to be a significant partner in his company. Mr. Bradford wanted to use my talents and my credentials for his personal gain. He would expect me to 'fluff' the people whenever it would be necessary for him and the company's benefit. It did not matter to him that the people who attended the seminar were sincerely looking for real answers to their real health insurance questions. Their time and my personal reputation was never a point of consideration from Mr. Bradfords' point of view.

I did sulk on the matter for a few months until I could regain my personal strength of positive thinking again.

The hard lesson I learned was that my true love for others comes with honor and respect; no fluff. And this will always be my genuine position in life. My desire to enjoy life is to have respect and peace for everyone I meet: To show genuine love for others.

CHAPTER 5 RECAP

<u>Enjoy Love & Peace with Family & Others</u>

- The positive attitude is love
- Positive people avoid negative people
- Time is the commodity of life.
- Enjoy your life one day at a time
- The benefits of a daily hug
- Have genuine love for others ((ACTUAL EVENT)

6
_____

REAL SELF LOVE

Accept yourself

Accepting yourself for who and what you are is one of your greatest personal assets. It is also the best place to start from when you are serious about changing your mindset.

Love yourself first for just who you are. Then begin your planning to bring about a better more positive lifestyle that gives real life changing benefits. Moving forward with a plan for a positive thinking mindset for your life requires total acceptance of who and what you are.

When we question some things about ourself such as," Why is my nose so small?" or "Why are my feet so big?" We can create a negative issue of dislike of ourself that we may never be able to mentally accept and overcome. And if you can't accept what you may consider imperfections or defaults about yourself, you will damage your ability to fully embrace a true love of self.

No one is perfect: period. And not one of us is expected to be perfect in any sense of understanding. It is important to accept this as a fact before you can truly know your self in the right terms of thinking positive about yourself.

To properly know who you are and what you are made of, honestly and faithfully identify the following:

- What are your prejudices? Are they based in fact or fiction?
- What are the virtues of life that you respect and give value to?
- What are the personality traits that encourage your negative thinking and inhibit your positive thinking thoughts?

Open the door to see the real person that you are by answering these questions honestly. A strong mental attachment to knowing yourself is to love yourself. Accept yourself for who and what you are without making excuses for any deficiencies you may feel you have. Respect yourself for who you are without restrictions.

Avoid self-criticism. Never say anything bad about yourself to anyone. There will always be someone else who will do that part for you. And sad to say, but I must say it because it is true: It is usually a family member or a close 'so-called' friend who trashes or belittles your good name.

Celebrate yourself when you achieve goals and celebrate yourself whenever you display resilience in the face of setbacks and adversities. Sometimes it's perfectly 'ok' to feel that you need and deserve a break today. Celebrate yourself! And once you have achieved a genuine love of self never doubt your abilities to succeed at whatever you desire to achieve. Whenever you are faced with any kind of challenge that appears to set you back, stop and think. Remind yourself that your self love is real. And no one can take your love of self away. It is your self love that drives your determination to succeed.

SELF PORTRAIT - the photographers lens

I share with you a beautiful self-expose process that I found rewarding that worked for me.

Whenever you experience an unexpected circumstance in your life's journey such as a job or career change, determine to take a closer look at yourself. Mentally hover outside of your body just long enough to envision looking at yourself. Or you can hire a professional photographer to do a self portrait photo shoot!

A photo shoot is a series of self portrait photos taken in several facial and body poses at different angles. By allowing the camera to see you in several different poses and angles it can reveal something about your appearance that you never saw before. After reviewing the photographers' work there should be two or more photos that captures an essence of you from your perspective views (ideas) of yourself.

"Over the course of the photo shoot drop the mask; the selfie-you. Allow yourself to be 'seen.' A good photographer can coach you. We are all uniquely beautiful and mysterious. There is no such thing as un-photogenic." These are the words of professional photographer, Nick Dantona. [*]

Make the opportunity to see yourself in a different light from a different angle. You will see and think of yourself with a different perspective.

---

[*] Nick Dantona Nashville, Tennessee Visit ndantona.com

It really works! I did it and found a new me. You will see several different images of yourself which you could have never imagined without the professional photographers' portrait lens. Take a good look at yourself!

Identity crisis - Who do you think you are

In the process of finding the real you, identify and define who and what you think you are.

We can defeat our demons only if we know who and where they are; hidden within our personality. And also possibly among our family and friends. Again, I sadly make this statement because this is the history of the world. Our betrayers in life will always be those who are closest to us. It's no fable or old wives tale that those who are closest to us are the ones who have the greatest opportunity to harm us: Because we will never allow our known enemies to get that close to us.

Find your demons wherever they are and cast them out as stepping stones to a better future.

To have true love of yourself (and you should) requires that you acknowledge:

- Who are you?
- What makes you who you are?
- What is your opinion of yourself?

Take an honest look within yourself and answer these questions with conviction to being totally truthful. Identify your naturally positive and sometimes negative instincts.

Here is an exercise to help you find some answers.

Arrange a lunch date with just one family member or a friend. Start a conversation with discussions on a variety of topics. Share each other's opinions with the intent to learn something new and different. Discuss the virtues of your positive views and attitudes versus your guests' views. Identify all negative and positive positions. Talk less and listen more. Listen for points of views that are different from your thinking. Take mental notes or written notes for later review and analysis. You will learn something about yourself if you are paying attention to the conversation.

Make it a point to repeat this type of socializing with other family members and friends: one on one only. Look to identify your positive and negative thinking thoughts in comparison to others. Over time, from these meetings you will see how to develop a framework for your positive thinking mindset; all based in who you are and how you may react in certain situations.

Make a list of the habits and routines that you experience everyday.

- Where do you go when you leave your house?
- What persons do you see on a regular basis?
- Who are the people in your circle of influence?

Make note of what topics you talk about and with whom.

Be specific here because this will tell you who influences and reinforces your positive and negative thoughts and ideas.

For sure we all have certain topics we discuss, only with certain people. What are the topics you talk about? Dig deep inside your mind searching for the thoughts you have about each one of your friends and associates. This exercise can help you identify the types of friends you keep; the people with whom you 'carousel,' go around with, in your life.

Once you can define yourself you will come to know who you are and what you are made of. This information will help you to see who and what influences your decision making.

How can you know yourself? Answer the question, "Who am I?" Identify what personality traits you may have inherited or created. Challenge yourself to create your own identifying questions. Creating your own questions will lead you to dig a little deeper into your soul. Within our soul is where our true personality exists.

Remember: This exercise is for your eyes only; so you can be completely honest with your answers.

Identify your personality.

I do… / I do not…

• respect authority

• love my Mother? Father? Siblings?

• respect my neighbor

• love my neighbor

• have empathy for people other than my family and friends

• care about other people

• fear strangers

• need friends

• believe in the Bible? Quran? Torah?

• believe in (a) God?

• believe in religion

• like people (Choose your color or ethnicity)

• like men / women

• love to win at everything

• hate to lose at anything

• care about winning or losing when playing games or sports

• respect others who are not like me or who do not look like me

I am... /I am not...

• a prejudice thinking person

• a racist thinking person

• a loving person

• considerate of others

• hopeful

• scared and fearful

Continue with your own items and questions until you become exhausted or run out of material to use.

This is a 'Personality Cheat Sheet' where you are allowed to feel and say whatever you want.

It is designed for your use only.

The answers you provide tells you and you alone where your positive and negative thoughts are coming from. When you have finished, compare the results with the social environment you live in. Some of your answers will be reflective of a universal attitude of popular thinking. Some of your responses may require more than a yes or no response.

Write out complete answers as much as possible. Do your best to qualify each one of your answers as a negative or a positive.

The sum total importance of this Personality Cheat Sheet is that you will get the chance to gather and record your thinking thoughts on a variety of human condition topics.

Completing this Personality Cheat Sheet gives you an opportunity to reveal hidden qualities in your personality: Positive and negative.

Don't be alarmed at any of your answers. Remember, this is for your eyes only.

If you do learn something about yourself that may be upsetting and cause you to feel anxious, talk to someone immediately. Don't be afraid to reach out for assistance if you feel unsure or uneasy about any of your answers.

The best time to tackle a problem issue is at first notice of the issue being a problem.

Take your time with this task. Add to it continuously until you feel it is complete. This task is truly... all about you.

ARE you a positive or negative person?

Why would I want to be positive everyday? Sounds a bit boring. Redundant even. "You're wrong!"

- Change your thinking.
- Change your mindset.
- Change your life.

Embrace the single idea that maintaining a positive attitude and outlook on life is beneficial to your mental and physical well being.

Is there a choice? Yes. You can choose to be negative or positive. "Can I be both negative and positive as it pleases me?" Yes. And my own experiences tell me most of us move between a negative and positive attitude without ever knowing it. We make our decisions based on the situation or circumstances at the moment void of the merits of creating a positive or negative outcome.

A real and true strength in all of life is the using, maintaining and sustaining a positive thinking attitude everyday. The positive attitude defeats the negative energy coming from the negative thinking society that we encounter everyday.

Also, positive thinking energy is in our DNA. It is easier and more productive to work with the positive energy you already have. You don't lose anything when you maintain a positive thinking mindset.

Most people are of a somewhat basic positive thinking mindset without ever realizing there is a choice. And this is because of the naturally positive thinking energy that is already written into our DNA.

So then what is positive and what is negative? To describe the negative we use the mathematical sign '-' which means to take away to reduce. Using the positive mathematical sign '+' means to add to increase. We do have a choice as to how we may desire to live our lives. Use the positive sign in your thinking for positive results.

Positive thinking people rule the World. Positive thinking is an attitude. And thinking positive and using a positive thinking mindset is a process that can be achieved by anyone. Although we are designed with a positive thinking energy source, it is our normal overthinking processes mixed with our cognitive distortions that incline us to accept many of the negative influences of our society. And these negatives that we accept give us more self-doubt causing low self-confidence, ultimately reducing our self-esteem.

There are those who would advise you to, *"Love your negatives.*

Embrace your negatives because negatives are a part of you." I disagree completely.

Negatives by definition are subtractions that take away. So don't waste your life embracing negatives when being completely receptive to your naturally given positive thinking energies offer the greatest benefits in life: A positive winning lifestyle.

Never embrace your negatives. Rise above the demons of your negative thinking. Overcome them and place them beneath you. Use your negative demons as stepping stones into a positive thinking mindset for your future! We were not designed or made with negatives. There is no such thing as negative energy DNA.

Our Creator has made us in His image. And there is nothing negative about Him or any of His creations. He did not make a negative living people.

But know that living life itself has created built-in negative demons everywhere and in everything we think and do.

Here are a few very popular negatives to let go of.

- Evil thinking - witchcraft
- Spiritism - Voodoo
- Hatefulness; prejudice
- Sinful living - sexual immorality
- To Lie, cheat, or deceive
- Murder, mayhem and to intentionally hurt and harm
- To whisper(signifying)
- To frighten intentionally
- To have no respect or empathy for the 'stranger'

And of course there are many more negatives too numerous to mention here.

Negatives by their own definition are minuses that say, 'take away.' Negatives are draining.

Positives by definition are pluses that say 'add on.' Positives are life sustaining.

Don't fear the process of developing a positive mindset. Engage it. Welcome the process step by step.

- Desire to be a positive thinking person.
- Make a daily plan/routine for coping with and removing negatives.
- Apply the plan of your design daily by using positive mindset affirmations.

Maintaining a positive attitude will improve your entire life. This improvement will be noticed in your healthier looking posture with a more upright walking style.

Generally positive thinking people 'walk tall' with their heads held up never looking down and with no slouching at any time. Imagine yourself each morning walking and talking with a positive attitude. Display your positive outlook for every day.

Whenever you experience an immediate energy surge of feeling confident know this as a sign to get engaged in doing some kind of positive physical activity. Go for walk, take a bike ride or get to the gym. Go on a date for a warm embrace; give a hug! You are experiencing an energy surge that needs some physical satisfaction. Now that you know what to do when that mood hits you...Go for it!

Issues. Problems. Attitudes. People will change and cause you to react. But react positively. This is life and things will happen to cause change. Don't be alarmed. This is life and things must happen. But you don't have to get bent out of shape or noticeably upset when things are not going your way. Your positive learning and instruction will teach you that all things must pass. The good and the bad must have their day. Your positive thinking mindset tells you to be patient, be firm and be ready. Through all of it stay positive, one day at a time always looking for the light at the end of each day. Whatever goodness comes into your life is meant for you. Whatever is for you, are waiting just for you to take. If you don't take the goodness that is meant for you it will just waste away because it has only your name on it. This is positive energy talk! Get what is yours. Now! Positively!

It is only one day at a time that we can experience actual life. Yesterday has passed. Tomorrow is the future. We have today to be thankful and grateful for. Live each day as it comes. This is the apex of life…living joyously one day at a time! Remember, it is all in your mind. And your real self love is in your DNA.

Have self-compassion in a big way

To be self-compassionate is to have empathy for yourself. Consider your self to be worthy of goodness, kindness and respect from everyone. Know that you are not a product of mistakes but a creation formed from an intelligent design by your Creator. Stay particularly aware of any and all negative thoughts. Negative thoughts easily turn into negative thinking. The patterns of negative thinking will often lead to negative actions.

Do not hold onto past regrets of what you should have, would have or could have done. View your entire past as stepping stones into your future. Look forward to accomplishing your future projects step by step one at a time.

Be kind to yourself. Make a vow to yourself that no setback will define you or keep you from your appointed goals.

Maintain a steadfast acceptance of the compassion you have for yourself. Being sincere in caring for yourself, significantly reduces overthinking, stress, needless worry and anxiety. Everyday, remind yourself that what is meant for you in your life is literally waiting for you.

Also, celebrate yourself privately. You don't need a crowd of friends to help you recognize your true inner growth. Your own self-celebrations are your acknowledgements of a job well done in reaching your goals. Remember to celebrate all of your self-achievements in your journey through life. Remind yourself that what is meant for you in your life is waiting for you.

SHARING the love

Acknowledge to yourself that you are a good person. Remind yourself to think good thoughts about yourself. And as hard as it may be, think good thoughts about others even when you believe they are not deserving of your good thoughts about them. Maintaining a good mental attitude that harbors no ill feelings against others is designed to help you. There's no negative overthinking thoughts when you don't hold grudges. Historical human psychology research tells us that when we think good of others and offer our forgiveness for trespasses committed against us, our personal stress levels are reduced. No overthinking stress.

Think right toward people. Smile and greet the stranger (be particular) with a cheerful acknowledgement of their presence. From the majority of your greeting presentations to strangers you will receive many positive responses.

If you know that you do not and cannot think good of all people because you harbor some reason to dislike or hate, know that this creates a mental conflict within you. And this conflict needs to be resolved before you will be able to mentally access the full strength of a positive thinking mindset that gives you true love of yourself.

When you sincerely explore all the possibilities of who you are you can then develop the ability to appreciate and love yourself for who and what you are. Self identification will show you where you fit in with family, friends, your neighborhood and society.

So go for it! Figure out who you are and then start to love yourself even more. It's ok. You can't give genuine love to someone else if you don't have genuine love for yourself.

Remember: You are a creation of God. Whether you accept this as fact or not this is the truth of life. We are all God's creations. And we are all the same human beings with the same positive energy DNA.

ABOVE ALL, love yourself

As the mind dictates we are allowed to do whatever it is we may we want to do. We do not and will not do something we truly do not want to do. Above all things love yourself.

As creations of God we are privileged to do whatever we want to do. And it is our Creators' love that provides for all of us. Even for those who don't want to believe in Him. He provides all the basic necessities we all need to live. No. He provides *everything* we all need to live. What an awesome God!

To enjoy a life worth living is to have real self-love with genuine self-compassion and a sincere display of honesty and gratitude.

Embrace your fears

During my teen years growing up I often had a reoccurring dream that would become a nightmare.

Initially I would pleasantly fall asleep and start dreaming about my love of flying like a bird in the sky. I would fantasize about flying high past the clouds. And then I would slowly swoop downward toward the peeks of the skyscrapers amongst all the tall buildings.

As I would start to descend my speed would uncontrollably accelerate to the point of free falling out of control. Now I'm spiraling downward head first at full speed for a deadly impact. Just before splashing dead to the ground I would immediately wake up in a relentless cold sweat with my heart beating in panic going a thousand miles a minute.

The dream would repeat itself at random for nearly a two year period during my early teen years. Whenever the dream would happen I would have no warning. Sometimes it would come just as I would fall asleep. But most times it was replayed toward the end of my sleep cycle just before morning wake up.

Toward the end of this two year period of these nightmare dreams I began to look for some kind of understanding of the dream. Even though I could not figure out why I was having the dream I rationalized that although the dream contained the fear of death, it was still just a dream. Because the dream contained a life and death component I reasoned that if I truly believed in God and if it was His desire to take me in this manner why should I fear His command in a dream? After having these particular thoughts I prayed that the next time the dream would occur I would try to allow the dream to complete itself with me falling to my death face first. I felt that if God was calling me in this way why should I refuse and continue to fight it? I would be very happy to be with God whenever He wanted me, however He would choose to take me. "Eureka!" With this understanding I had no more fear of the dream. I rejoiced and felt good about my decision and said to myself, "Bring on the dream!"

The next time the nightmare dream did occur I quickly remembered my prayers and discussions I had with God about the dream. This time when the dream progressed with me flying amongst the clouds I could feel a broad smile on my face as I began to descend among the skyscrapers. I remember a feeling of happiness and relief that 'it' was going to be over; no more nightmare. But I never went into a free fall to crash to ground to my death. In this dream I simply continued to fly. When I did wake up that morning all I remembered was smiling in my dream. My nightmare would come to an end with me not making a landing at all.

And to this day more than thirty years later I still dream of flying high amongst the clouds without ever making a landing! I embraced my fear of falling to my death. And on the strength of my prayers I have learned to have no fear of falling; or failing or dying.

Today I have no fears in my life. What I learned from this experience has helped me to be who and what I am today. I have come to know myself as a creation, a child of God who is in His hands eternally. In Jesus name I pray.

Have love of yourself. You are all you have. It is all about you…and your Creator. And He says…Love, eternally.

CHAPTER 6 RECAP

Have Real Love of self

- Accept yourself
- Self portrait - the photographers lens

- Identity crisis - Who do you think you are
- Are you a positive or negative person?
- Have self-compassion in a big way
- Sharing the love
- Above all, love yourself
- Embrace your fears (ACTUAL EVENT)

PERSONAL HAPPINESS EVERYDAY

Change your mindset change your life

The positive thinking mindset will tell you that even in a bad situation there is something positive to learn from the experience. This is the essence of a positive thinking mindset. You know you may not be able to solve all your problems but you maintain an optimistic belief that the possibilities exist that you can solve all your problems. With a positive thinking mindset you learn to accept whatever life brings because you are doing your best to be prepared for the challenges of life.

You are constantly aware and consistently open to learning how and when to use your positive instincts in all situations.

A positive thinking mind is always learning:

- When to be quiet, laid back and reflective when a 'no response' is the best solution in an argumentative conversation.

- To practice being humble, but intuitively assertive in negotiating situations.
- To have great patience yet demanding if necessary when settling tense disputes.
- To show humility for others; family and friends and the stranger.
- To talk less and listen more intently especially when involved in emotional situations.
- To be mindful of the natural tendency for negative overthinking; averting needless worries.
- To work tirelessly to eliminate most, if not all cognitive distortions.

When you put in the sincere effort needed to think positive your results will be positive.

STRENGTHEN your positive mindset

Each morning as you get up from your bed to start a new day, look directly into your mirror. Look into your eyes and remind yourself who you are. Do this every morning for a planned starting point to each day. Make serious eye contact with your mirror image and engage your positive thinking mind by reciting your planned morning affirmations.

Schedule each day with a 'to do list' and commit to getting it done. Be confident and know that you are in charge of your life and in control of all the moving parts. Whenever it is wise and prudent to take a day off from work, take the day off!

Use the following guidelines for your daily activities.

- Have an exercise routine for each day: even if it is just a brisk walk. Any type of aerobic exercise that gets the heart pumping for a minimum 15 minutes is adequate.
- Make healthy food choices all day. Remind yourself that you are determined to eat a healthy foods diet. Never give up on finding every way possible to eat healthy foods. If you do have a setback, remain calm and quietly start again.
- No alcohol. Reduce your daily consumption of all alcohol products. Alcohol pleasures the mind but destroys the body. Tell yourself repeatedly that the body does not like or need alcohol. If you do continue with your alcohol beverage pleasures, reduce your daily intake. Accept the true facts about alcohol beverages with an open mind: Alcohol in all forms is a poison to the body. Notice how one alcohol drink(beer) affects the mind. Most people say "It relaxes me." But alcohol to the brain is not a relaxer, it'a stimulant to the brain and a poison to the internal organs. We don't need alcohol at all.
- Avoid negative situations and all people you may know who have negative attitudes and opinions. This will be hard at first but stay focused to accomplish this goal.
- Keep company with only positive thinking people because they will influence and encourage you to find your own ways of positive thinking behaviors. Think of yourself as the positive side of the magnet looking for positive people to attract.
- Stay completely aware of your surroundings at all times. One way to 'fine tune' your mental focus is to exercise your eyes. Open wide and focus your vision on a distant object. Hold this focus for at least 10 seconds. Now refocus on an object that's closer to you. Hold for ten seconds. This exercise has the power to help you regain your present moment's reality. Repeat this eye exercise at least three

times throughout the day. It will help you to re-focus
mentally and visually.

- Ask yourself, "What are the negatives in my life that I
  should get rid of? What are the positives I need to bring
  into my life?
- Start living in every moment of your life. Smell the
  roasting of the coffee. Experience the touch of the silky
  soft pedals of a rose. Look up to the stars at night more
  often.
- Get in touch with nature. Walk along the beach at sunrise
  or sunset. Take a nature walk in the forest or in the park.
- Affirm / Pray / meditate, daily. It gives you strength and
  courage to move on in spite of your problems and missteps.

Throughout the day do the following:

- Mentally focus on the good things of life.
- Treat yourself with respect and kindness all day long.
- Look forward to giving a hand to a neighbor, friend or a
  stranger (be selective here).
- If you make the slightest mistake at anytime during the
  day, forgive yourself immediately and forget about it.
- Whatever mistake or error you do make always look for the
  positive benefit. Let go of the memory of the error and
  move on.
- Remind yourself that each new day brings new blessings.
  It's True!

Each day, while doing your daily activities quietly recite your positive affirmations. This process encourages you mentally to get close
and personal with your feelings.

Bring peace to your everyday

However we think we feel has a definite impact on how we actually feel. The benefits of thinking with a positive mindset everyday will increase your happiness everyday allowing you to enjoy the following benefits.

- You become more aware and attentive to your physical appearance with the desire to look your best at all times.
- Just from thinking more positively about yourself your body begins to develop a stronger immune system.
- You will record a lower blood pressure reading which translates into reduced risks of heart disease.
- Being in a positive state of mind you will experience less worry and less stress. This wards off any threats of anxiety.
- You become more attractive physically and mentally in relationships. And your attraction is made stronger because of clearer understandings of the relationships.

A positive thinking mindset teaches you how to develop and design your own coping mechanisms to better handle the daily challenges of life itself. As you become more confident in your positive thinking you gain courage to take on more achievement risks thus by increasing your chances of reaching your goals much faster. But take it slow. Over confidence and cockiness can send you backwards in your journey.

Whenever you are being confronted with a negative thinking situation immediately identify it as negative thoughts and start to apply the following positive thinking.

- Focus your thinking thoughts on one or more of the positives things that have happened in your life. This

change of focus will remove the negative thoughts
immediately.

- Begin a new train of thought patterns eliminating the old
  way of thinking. Clear your thinking and say to yourself
  that you must change your thinking of negative thoughts to
  positive thoughts.

Stay determined and motivated to maintain a positive thinking
mind. In a short period of time your naturally positive mental
instincts will take over and help you in every way: Because that's
how positive thinking energy works!

Your naturally positive energy DNA takes action by immediately
responding to your mental request.

Always challenge your negative thoughts as to whether or not they
are valid thoughts worthy of your attention and use. Negative
thinking thought patterns is where the potential exists to create
demons in your thinking.

To dismiss a negative thought permanently and to keep it from
randomly coming back you must replace it with a positive thought.
And in most cases the negative thought will be eliminated never to
return on its own accord.

Test yourself. Think of a recent negative thought you had. Now
simply repeat the opposite positive thought at least 3 times . Feel
the positive energy surge? When you have mentally replaced a
negative thought with a positive thought, the negative thought will
not come back. You will have to mentally summon the negative
thought to come back. And if you don't replace the negative thought
with a positive thought the negative thought will find a place to
hibernate somewhere in your mind to reoccur into your thought
patterns at its own discretion.

Use the positive process to remove your negative thoughts permanently for a happier more positive lifestyle.

Share your appreciation for others

During my 15 plus years in real estate as a real estate agent and real estate broker, I was also a rental property owner. Throughout those years I helped many people find a place to call home.

As a building contractor and property manager I did my best to create nice, clean and updated homes for their comfort. And the majority of them showed their appreciation for my efforts by routinely paying their rent on time.

In all my time of 7+ years renting properties, I recall processing no more than two full rental evictions where a Sheriff had to come and physically remove the tenant. My overall benefits in the apartment management business was financially rewarding and mentally insightful. Nearly all of the tenants were good hearted respectfully people who were very kind to me. Through these experiences I gained the knowledge of having a better understanding of people in general.

What I learned has given me wisdom to believe in the average person. When you give someone an honest and decent chance to prove themselves to be worthy, most people will show their appreciation by keeping their word to honor their commitments. Expect the best, not the worst from people. Having an overall general faith in people will definitely help to keep your stress levels down.

Offer first, your positive attitude and that will bring out their positive responses to you. Everyday, bring out the natural positivity in others with your positive thinking attitude.

And this is how you will find your happiness…everyday!

. . .

Everything in it's proper place works fine

True happiness is a desired personal experience. It is in our soul where we experience the true feelings of happiness. We are contented, delighted, pleased and feel glad with ourselves over a particular thing, a person or an event.

A long lasting happiness is based in the good we think of ourselves and what we think of others. With a positive thinking mindset you can have the opportunities to experience happiness everyday. As life comes with it's ups and downs where nothing is perfect, you have to accept as fact that some days will be harder than others to get through.

It is a lifelong journey developing and nurturing a positive thinking mind that produces the benefits of happiness everyday. And because it is a journey, part of the development process requires you to stop along the way at each achievement point and celebrate yourself by mentally and emotionally saying "I did it!"

With a positive thinking mindset everyday happiness is possible just like the running of a well maintained furnace that has the potential to run forever: If you maintain it. Accept as fact that changing the way you think to a positive thinking mindset will change your life. All according to God's plan with everything in its proper place everything works fine.

Good memories create happy tomorrows

In times of stress and sorrow if we can recall good memories from our past we have the chance to create a more pleasant future.

When we have to experience the passing of a loved one we grope for the memories of good times shared with them. The good memories tend to make the present loss more palatable.

Everyday do whatever you can to create good memories for your future. I share with you an actual event. The names are factious but the event is real.

While working at the *Half Sandwich Cafe* in Miami, Florida as a short order cook, I would often hear Luis my boss, the chef and owner of the cafe talk 'down' to his wife Angeline, the dining room manager and cashier. Angeline was about 37 years old. She had a slim to skinny build with a medium stature of just 5 feet. Luis, 42 years old, was slightly tall, just over 6 feet and a bit robust. They were a working compliment to each other. Both were very capable of being fast with their hands and agile on their feet when needed. In the fast food service business speed with agility is mandatory for success.

They had a 6 year old son Antony, an only child who all would agree was spoiled rotten; just the way Luis and Angeline wanted him to be.

After two week of working at the *Half Sandwich Cafe* I witnessed Luis being rude to Angeline in front of the customers. He literally went on a 'tear' talking down to his wife in the heat of a busy lunch service. Soon, I became aware of the fact that Luis was rude to Angeline more regularly than not. It seemed like every other day of the week Luis would ridicule Angeline during the lunch service. Everyday became a hard days' work at the cafe for me. I was not happy to hear Luis talk so harshly to his wife. Now I come to work everyday feeling sad repeating to myself "There is no joy in Mudville. There is no joy in Mudville." *

---

* Reference made to famous poem, "Casey at the Bat" by Ernest Lawrence Thayer.

Then one day when Luis's behavior was just so horribly rude to Angeline, I asked him if he and I could sit down together and have a talk after lunch service. From the quizzical expression on his face I could tell he had no idea as to why I wanted to talk with him. As soon as lunch service was over, the kitchen cleaned and made ready for tomorrows' lunch service, Luis and I sat down for our talk. Without any hesitation I immediately said to him that if he continues to be so rude to his wife in front of the customers and me, that I would not remain here to work for him. He gave no response. For the next few minutes Luis looked away from me with a blank stare towards the floor. I broke the silence by asking him *"When was the last time the two of you went out for a nice dinner?"* His response was *"I can't remember."* This would be the first time I interjected myself into Angeline and Luis's personal life. And it was because his negative behavior was affecting my positive thinking lifestyle.

That evening while I sat home I began to think a bit more about Luis and Angeline. I had met Luis when I job interviewed at his cafe for the short order cook position a month earlier. He hired me on the spot at the interview. He would later tell me that during the kitchen-prep test part of the interview it was my 'fast hands' performance that he liked about me. *" You got to have fast hands and think on your feet to be a good short order cook, so I hired you, "* is what he said to me. That night, I scratched my brain thinking, wanting to find a way to help Luis and Angeline. But what could I do? My positive thinking thoughts started percolating.

"Eureka!" An observation I made was that Luis and Angeline worked together all day in the restaurant starting at 5:30 in the morning serving breakfast and lunch until 3:00 in the afternoon, Monday through Friday. Luis is the chef, the main cook who

Hope turns to despair.

manages the kitchen with a couple of kitchen hands. Angeline is the hostess, dining room manager and cashier managing a waitstaff of 3. The restaurant would serve 75-100 customers daily for breakfast and lunch, Monday through Friday only: No Saturdays or Sundays.

In my overall thinking of Luis and Angeline I calculated that the majority of their lives being together was working in the cafe throughout the week. Luis had mentioned to me previously that the weekends, Saturdays and Sundays were primarily preparation times for the cafe: They would go food shopping to wholesale grocery stores and farmers markets.

But Luis's rudeness to his wife did not stop. It happened again. He was so brutal to Angeline I asked him once again if I could talk to him after lunch service. This time I asked that Angeline be there also. After the lunch service, we all three sat down together. I explained to Luis for the second time that if he continues to belittle his wife in front of the customers like he did today, I would simply walk out of the restaurant during the lunch service. This time he responded to me. First, he rightfully apologized to his wife and then said to me; *"I don't mean to be rude I just can't control myself when I see something is being done the wrong way."* And then he said in a soft voice with a teardrop in his eye that he loves and adores his wife; he exclaimed, *"She is my life."*

What I had been witnessing while working at the cafe, was a marriage made on working. They lived and breathed the business. Everything they did was all built around the business; the *Half Sandwich Cafe*. My observations and Luis's explanations told me that they had no memories! They had no recall of sharing 'good times' with each other. Their lives together appeared to be void of any emotional affection of touching and hugging with tender kisses.

"Luis" I yelled. *"You have no memories! The two of you are working so hard for the cafe that you have neglected taking time to*

make real memories of celebrating each other, sharing good times together. It is our memories of positive times that will carry us through the hard work and the harsh times. You guys have no positives to recall! You have no memories of having a good time for your lives."

I went on to say that when times are tough or simply not looking so good, you need to have an anchor, a place in your mind that you can go to and get some renewed positive energy. It is in our memories where we find the help to get through the tough times. If you have no memories of good times in your past you are all set up for a tough future. And it will continue to be a tough future until you do something to change the cycle. I said to both of them; *"Go out and make some good memories! Enjoy your life! Find a way to do something you both can enjoy other than working!"* This is what I told Luis and Angeline, almost in a demanding voice.

The very next day after the lunch rush was over Luis and Angeline asked me to come have a coffee and sit with them. As we all sat down Luis then asked me if I would help to run the cafe for two weeks. He went on to say that he and Angeline had a very emotional talk late into the night and came up with the decision to take a vacation. In a very loud and excited voice, Luis said *"I am taking my beautiful, loving and devoted wife to Las Vegas!"*

When they returned two weeks later you could see 'Lovebirds' in the air around their heads. I heard no more discouraging remarks out of Luis. Not even a mean word to the kitchen hands! It seems as though everyday happiness at the cafe was about to become a reality. There will be 'Joy in Mudville' after all!

What Luis needed, he got. He needed to see the world again without the cafe. He needed to see a reality that exists outside of himself and to acknowledge his wife as more than just an employee or business partner. He did these things. Surprisingly to me he did these things immediately. With a positive attitude he accepted my observations and followed up with positive actions delivering all positive results!

Luis also learned to create his own happiness. Because their trip to Las Vegas went so well they made future plans to return to Vegas every six months, if possible. Luis had come to a realization that it is important to be positive and take positive actions to make loving memories with his family; just for memory sake!

When we take the time to mentally visualize the successes of our past accomplishments we are energized to have the courage to take on new challenges. And we truly look forward to succeeding again and again. We all must remember that we can't live in the past. It is our future that awaits us. And the elusive present time is our actual life.

In your present moments take the time to make good memories for your future. When you need comfort and reassurance let it come from within as memories from your past. With good memories from our past we can plan how to have a better more enjoyable future; everyday.

CHAPTER 7 RECAP

Personal Happiness Everyday

- Change your mindset change your life
- Strengthen your positive mindset
- Bring peace to your everyday
- Share your appreciation for others
- Everything in it's proper place works fine
- Good memories create happy tomorrows (ACTUAL EVENT)

CONCLUSION

You are who you think you are...

And when you think positive thoughts about yourself, you will generally make positive decisions that generate your positive behaviors.

The following facts identify positive thinking people.

• Positive thinking people have a true unselfish love of self that helps to create their genuine peace of mind.

• Constantly being in a positive thinking state of mind brings peace and quiet that comforts the soul, giving a feeling of life satisfaction.

• They are the ones who continually make real accomplishments and achievements toward their desired goals. These accomplishments strengthen and reinforce their self confidence.

• Forever on a journey through life seeking and acquiring knowledge from continuously reading and exploring new ways of thinking.

• They remain focused seeking knowledge and acquiring wisdom sharing love and happiness with family and friends, everyday!

As a society...

we can be easily defined as a massive ball of confusion. Yet everyday we navigate our lives through the traffic of negative thought patterns that are connected to our cognitive distortions creating a brew of harmful and needless overthinking. Yes, a massive ball of confusion we are.

But the positive mind finds pathways to positive power for logical reasoning and celebrations of the positive achievements that we accomplish each day.

"Although the mind creates all of your problems it is your mind that is also the only thing in charge of solving them." *

Your positive thinking mindset may not win at every outing. But facing each days' challenges with a positive thinking attitude will definitely place the 'odds' of having a great day in your favor. Be fearlessly courageous to persevere in your positive thinking. We have all the positive thinking tools we need to succeed in life. Practice keeping your mind clear of distortions. *"Don't carry your positive thinking tools around in a tool bag that has holes in it allowing negatives to seep in."* BRYANSCOTT PARKER

As a forward thinking society...

we must be destined to heal ourselves through naturally positive energy applications. It is hugely beneficial for each of us as individuals and collectively, to embrace goodness, truth and the righteous side of the law. We must vehemently reject the dishonest behaviors

---

* Excerpt from OVERTHINKING? 7 Steps to finding Peace from Overthinking Stress, Anxiety and Worry, Bryanscott Parker

of all liars and deceivers who use negative ideas and negative thinking as a power base to win us over for their own personal agendas. Over time we will destroy ourselves through hate, jealousy, and deceit. A house divided will not stand. We are greater than such a perilous end. We must repel our negatives.

Acquire the knowledge of thinking positive everyday. Enjoy the wisdom of living a long and happy life: Because you can. Allow 'The Art of Positive Thinking' to activate the positive energy written into your DNA assigned to you at birth.

Enjoy the 7 most powerful benefits of thinking positive everyday. It is all in your mind.

Think positive because positive thinking energy is in your DNA. You can't leave home without it!

GLOSSARY

This Glossary has been added because it has been my life experiences telling me that a read along word guide can be most beneficial when reading and studying new self-help material. It is provided to assist you in having full access to the understanding of all the terms and expressions used in the writing of this book.

For the young readers who are eager to learn and grow, this book is a collection of beautiful and descriptive word choices to enhance their learning and speaking vocabulary.

For more word choices in this genre of self-help, visit the Glossary in the 1st book of The Positive Mind book series;

OVERTHINKING? 7 Steps to finding Peace from Overthinking Stress, Anxiety and Worry.

A

acuity sharpness or keenness of thought: mental, visual

accomplishment something done admirably or creditably

affirmation the act of alarming; a positive assertion

agile able to move quickly and easily

agility the quality or state of being agile

alleviate to partially remove or correct

alienated made to feel isolated or estranged.

altruistic having or showing an unselfish concern for the welfare of others

ascribe to refer to a supposed cause

assertive having, showing a confident personality

aspects a particular part or feature of something

attributes a quality or feature regarded as a characteristic

avert to see coming and ward off

B

Bias an inclination of temperament or outlook especially: a personal and sometimes unreasoned judgment: prejudice

C

cavalier given to offhand dismissal of important matters

caveat a modifying or cautionary detail

circadian rhythms which refers to the inherent cycle of about 24 hours that appears to control various biological processes, such as sleep, wakefulness, and digestive activity

conflict to be different, opposed, or contradictory

consummate complete in every detail

conundrum an intricate and difficult problem

D

deity the rank or essential nature of a god

delineation the act of outlining or representing something

detrimental obviously harmful; damaging

discretion individual choice or judgment

E

essential of the utmost importance : basic, necessary

F-G

grope to feel about blindly or uncertainly in search

H-I

immense marked by greatness especially in size or degree

inebriated exhilarated or confused by or as if by alcohol

inhibit a: to hold in check, restrain;

irrational not rational, lacking usual normal mental clarity

J-K

karma the force generated by a person's actions held in Hinduism and Buddhism

keen intellectually alert :having or characteristic of a quick penetrating mind

L-M

monotony tedious, sameness

N

nuance a subtle distinction or variation

O

obtuse a subtle distinction or variation

optimism an inclination to put the most favorable construction upon actions and events or to anticipate the best possible outcome

P

palatable agreeable or acceptable to the mind

petrified overwhelmingly fearful; rendered motionless

poignant designed to make an impression: being to the point

prattle to utter or make meaningless sounds or conversation

proclivity an inclination or predisposition toward

promulgate to make (an idea, belief, etc.) known to many

Q

quipped a clever usually taunting remark; witty

quizzical expressive of puzzlement, curiosity, or disbelief

R

redundant a: exceeding what is necessary or normal. b: characterized by or containing an excess specifically using more words than necessary

replicate duplicate, repeat

repressed characterized by restraint

S

solace to give comfort to in grief or misfortune

stamina the bodily or mental capacity to sustain a prolonged stressful effort or activity

surmise a thought or idea based on scanty evidence

T

tangent an abrupt change of course

tenacious not easily pulled apart; persistent

tenets a principle, belief generally held to be true

U- V

vicarious experienced or realized through imaginative or sympathetic participation

vista a distant view through or along an avenue or opening

void containing nothing

W-X-Y-Z

RESOURCES

OVERTHINKING? 7 Steps to finding Peace from Overthinking Stress, Anxiety & Worry

(2023) Millennium Publishing, LLC

"Thinking is fundamental. Change your thinking, change your mindset."

author: Bryanscott Parker. bryanscottparker.com

Thrilling New Evidence Suggests Earth's Life Came from Space.

(March 21, 2023) popularmechanics.com

author: Jackie Appel

15 Cognitive Distortions to Blame for Negative Thinking.

(January 11, 2022) PsychCentral.com.

authors: Sandra Silva; Medically reviewed by Karin Geop.PsyD Casablanca.

All of the bases in DNA and RNA have now been found in meteorites

(April 26, 2022) sciencenews.org

author: Liz Kruesi

10 Health Benefits of Hugging, backed by Science

(March 26, 2020) mindbodygreen.com

author: Ashley Uzer, MBA; Medical reviewer: Bindiva Gandhi, M.D.

Relentless Optimism: How a Commitment to Positive Thinking Changes Everything

(2017) Shamrock New Media

"This book will show you just how powerful a positive attitude can be and it will teach you how to use positive thinking to make your biggest dreams come true."

author: Darrin Donnelly

The Power of Positive Thinking

(2015) Simon & Schuster

"This book is written with the sole objective of helping the reader achieve a happy, satisfying, and worthwhile life."

author: Norman Vincent Peale

The Motivation Manifesto

(2014) Hay House LLC

Excerpt from Summary: *"Recalling the revolutionary voices of the past that chose freedom over tyranny, Bouchard - at times poetic yet always fierce - motivates us to free ourselves from fear and take back our lives once and for all."*

Author: Brendon Burchard

How Successful People Think

(2009) Center Street

From the publisher: *"Become a better thinker through practical and actionable steps to help you reach a new level personally and professionally."*

author: John C. Maxwell

Make Today Count

(2008) Center Street

From the publisher: *"Readers will learn how to make decisions on important matters and apply those decisions daily to put them on a path to more successful, productive and fulfilling lives."*

author: John C. Maxwell

The Magic of Thinking Big

(1987) Reprinted. Simon & Schuster

"Those who believe they can move mountains, do. Those who believe they can't, cannot. Belief triggers the power to do."

author: David J. Schwartz,

Knowledge and Decisions

(1980) Basic Books

Excerpt from Preface

"The analysis begins with one of the most severe constraints facing human beings in all societies and throughout history-inadequate knowledge for making decisions that each individual and every organization nevertheless has to make, in order to perform the tasks that go with living and achieve the goals that go with being human."

author: Thomas Sowell

ABOUT THE AUTHOR

Visit - Bryanscottparker.com

Utilizing years of experience as an insurance broker and a real estate broker in Connecticut and Massachusetts, Bryanscott Parker developed a readers' 'Question/Answer' column in a local newspaper. The column was titled,

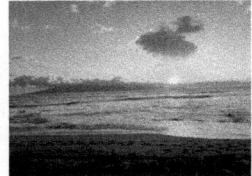

   'This House is For Sale. Let's Talk Real Estate with Bryanscott
   Parker."

The column was designed to provide first-time homebuyers with positive information on making their house purchase. In the column he would answer the readers' questions about buying their first home, obtaining the proper home insurance, working with contractors and seeking competent legal advice for their closings. Bryanscott was sharing his knowledge of real estate and insurance to those who needed positive guidance at a critical time - owning their first home.

And today, he is happily retired living his long awaited desires to write and write with positive compassionate care in the genre of self-help: To help everyone.

amazon.com/author/bryanscottparker52

linkedin.com/in/Bryanscott-parker-2465b1284